The Use of Herbal Remedies in the Treatment of Pain

Natural Pain Management & Herbal Remedies as Complementary Medicines.

Guy Chamberland, M.Sc., Ph.D., Herbalist

Disclaimer

Prior to taking any new herbal products/supplements, always check with your health-care practitioner.

Edited by: Ann Westlake, Writer's Cramp Editing Consultants.

Publisher: CuraPhyte Technologies Inc

ISBN 978-0-9877839-0-5

DEDICATION

To my wife, Céline, who gave me the opportunity to learn and practice herbology, and to my four daughters Elodie, Min Jee, Clara and Laura-Marie.

TABLE OF CONTENTS

FOREWORD

by Bryce Wylde

According to the National Institutes of Health (NIH), the annual cost of chronic pain in the United States alone is estimated to be about $100 billion. Most people have pain that can't be traced to a cause, such as fractures, infections, cancer, or significant changes that show up in tests or on imaging studies like MRI's and CT scans. A lot of pain arises from abusing the body mechanically, emotionally, and especially nutritionally. Millions of people in North America are overweight and underactive. Many have poor mobility and experience chronic pain. Pain itself fosters further inactivity. A massive percentage of the sedentary population in North America accounts, by in large, for the global obesity epidemic. Most of these people are in pain. Developed countries spend huge amounts of money on mechanical, electrical, and physical aids to accommodate those in pain thereby removing the need for movement, exercise, and activity. Inevitably obesity is on the rise leading to increased incidences of heart disease, diabetes, and cancer, as well as a plethora of other health concerns which plague our modern society.

If you look at the numbers, it becomes quite obvious that many people need help first to get out of pain so that they can then become more active. But when it comes to conventional pain management, mainstream medical treatment is too narrowly focused on the use of non-steroidal anti-inflammatory drugs (or NSAIDS), such as Aspirin, Advil, and Ibuprofen. These drugs can be effective in the short term, but they are also the *leading* cause of death due to drugs! Most people have no idea how dangerous these drugs are, popping them daily without considering long term effects. Since many of them can be bought over the counter without a prescription, the average person considers them harmless. The good news is that there are far safer and more effective approaches.

About 2000 BC, it was common place to hear "Eat this herb." Then circa 1000 AD, you might have heard, "That herb is heathen. Here, say this prayer." Sometime later around 1850 AD, "That prayer is superstition. Here, drink this potion." Not too long ago somewhere about 1940 AD you may have heard, "That potion is snake oil. Here, swallow this pill." More recently, around 1985 AD, it was common to hear, "That pill is ineffective. Here, take this antibiotic." It is now the year 2012, and more and more often we are hearing, "That antibiotic doesn't work. Here, eat this herb." It seems that we have come full circle!

Now enter Dr. Guy Chamberland, M.Sc., Ph.D., and Herbalist. Today, it is quite common to hear Guy say, "That pain medication doesn't work. Here, eat this herb."

Dr. Chamberland's suffering from lower back pain, and the excruciating pain were treated with a drug regimen. The side effects and alternative treatments, such as epidural injections of anesthetics and corticosteroids, only caused partial pain relief but also caused many other side effects. Pharmaceutical intervention was unsuccessful. His drug treatment was soon replaced by herbal remedies where he was able to obtain adequate pain relief.

While I personally have never experienced chronic pain, I am of the opinion that "an ounce of prevention is worth a pound of cure." I met up and consulted with Dr. Chamberland just prior to what would be one of the most challenging adventures of my life. This particular bucket list item had me convinced that in order to succeed, I needed to avoid succumbing to pain. I also intended to do my best to prevent injury and any long term repercussions. It was the summer of 2011 when I had decided to climb Mount Kilimanjaro – the highest mountain peak in Africa. Thanks in part to some of Dr. Chamberland's herbal formulas and a lot of will power, I was indeed successful. Over the course of the climb, I slept like a log and remained pain free.

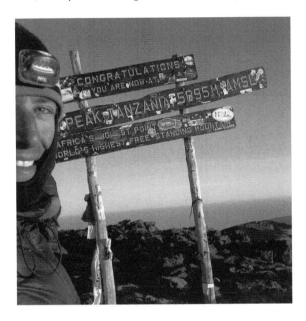

Dr. Chamberland has devoted his life to the field of herbal medicine and published authoritative texts on the subject. This book, *The Use of Herbal Remedies in the Treatment of Pain,* will inform patients and mainstream doctors in a new area of health care - one in which non-physicians have also emerged as health-care providers. It is also designed to offer the average person a wide range of natural choices in managing pain. It introduces a natural, herbal therapeutic approach that mimics the pharmaco-logical basis of how drugs are used to relieve pain.

Aside from the wonderful easy to understand lexicon of herbs found in this book, you will also learn the importance of cleansing, detoxification, repair, weight loss, regeneration, nutrition and physical activity in context of pain management. Dr. Chamberland's approach allows people with chronic pain - but without an extensive anatomical and physiological knowledge - to successfully help themselves.

The use of well-studied herbal remedies as a first line therapy can dramatically reduce the need for pharmaceutical and surgical interventions in anybody with pain. Read, study, and follow Dr. Chamberland's advice in this book and it will change your life for the better.

Here is to *you* becoming pain free!
Bryce Wylde

INTRODUCTION

Chamberland was first introduced to Chinese herbal medicine in 1990. This launched his interest in herbal medicine, and over the years he studied the pharmacology of many herbs.

Based on his experience working on complex pharmaceutical products, he was invited to present at the FDA Public Hearing on Regulation of Combination Products (http://www.fda.gov/CombinationProducts/MeetingsConferencesWorkshops/ucm133825.htm). Subsequently he wrote a chapter entitled *"Developing Drug-Device Combination Products with Unapproved Components"* for the textbook **Clinical Evaluation of Medical Devices**, edited by Becker, Karen M. and Whyte, John J., Humana Press, 2006.

In 2007 Chamberland began studying the additive and synergistic effects obtained when combining plant extracts. His interest in herbal pain management began early in 2007 after suffering from a L4-L5 disc hernia. The symptoms consisted of pain radiating from the lower back all the way to the tip of the toes, pain-induced insomnia, lower leg muscle cramps, and numbness on the surface of the skin of the right thigh. Pain relief was obtained by taking Dilaudid®, Naprosyn®, and Flexeril®. The undesirable side effects, including drowsiness, loss of concentration, etc, prevented him from continuing his scientific research. Alternatives, such as epidural injections of anaesthetics and corticosteroids, only caused partial pain relief but caused facial flushing, severe hypertension and aggressiveness. The lack of pharmaceutical drugs that could relieve the pain and also allow him to actively work as a scientist was what motivated his research into the development of herbal based remedies for pain. During very infrequent episodes of severe pain, herbs were combined with drugs in a complementary approach to minimize the use of narcotics and muscle relaxants and obtain adequate pain relief.

In 2009 Chamberland founded a company called CuraPhyte Technologies Inc (www.curaphyte.com; www. enteriphyte.com) that specializes in the development and commercialization of evidence-based herbal remedies. The company has two major axes of activities: one devoted to commercializing quality products for patient self-care lines, and the other devoted to commercializing professional product lines and working closely with health practitioners to further understand the treatment of pain with herbal remedies.

Chamberland has completed training as a natural health practitioner, bioenergetics practitioner, chartered herbalist, Master Herbalist thesis and in herbal prescriptions. Through his continued research in herbal science, he has become an expert in herbal pain management.

Chapter 1
A SIMPLIFIED LOOK AT PAIN KILLING DRUGS

This chapter provides a simplified explanation of some of the key pharmaceutical drugs used to relieve pain. (The use of herbal remedies complementary to these drugs is explained in Chapter 4.)

Complementary medicine is the use of both conventional medicine and alternative-natural medicines concurrently to obtain a safer and more effective therapy for the patient. Alternative-natural medicines can be added to the treatment by the physician to reduce the dosages of the pharmaceutical drug to avoid undesirable side effects in the patient, or simply to increase the therapeutic effectiveness of the therapy. Van Wyk and Wink (2010) described the use of Stinging nettle (Urtica dioica) for its anti-inflammatory properties as a complement to that of non-steroidal anti-inflammatory drugs (NSAIDs) in the treatment of arthritis. By adding Stinging nettle to the therapy, the physician was able to obtain more anti-inflammatory activity and avoid raising the dosage level of the NSAID.

Other key therapeutic aspects of pain management, such as sleep, exercise and nutrition are not discussed in this chapter. Since pain may prevent you from falling asleep or from having a restful sleep, your physician may prescribe pharmaceutical sleeping aids. Weight loss and exercise may also be part of the physician's therapeutic program to help you recover. For example, excessive body weight puts a lot more weight on a knee joint, and this excess pressure on the joint will contribute to the degree of pain. Obesity is also a contributing factor to osteoarthritis because of the extra weight on the joints.

In the case of fibromyalgia, numerous studies have shown that restful sleep is a key element to the recovery of the patient. Some of the studies demonstrated reduction in pain associated with patients obtaining restful sleep. It is also important for patients with fibromyalgia to exercise despite the fatigue. Exercise brings multiple benefits to the patient ranging from stimulating the immune system, relieving stress, stimulating the production of endorphins, to increasing endurance. Exercising does not mean becoming a professional athlete. It means beginning with simple changes, such as walking for 30 minutes three days a week, or other gentle exercise such as swimming, and with time slowly increasing the intensity and amount of exercise.

Note:

This chapter presents some of the side effects that are reported for the pharmaceutical drug. The reader needs to understand that these single synthetic molecules are usually powerful pharmacological agents and have provided very good pain relief to many patients. Some people are more sensitive than others to the effects of these drugs, and others are simply looking for a natural remedy. Many people take these pharmaceutical drugs and do not experience any of the side effects described below. In some cases, people initially experience undesirable effects but, over time, their body becomes able to process the drug and the side effects disappear. You should speak to your physician about complementary medicine, if you are a patient that experiences some of the undesirable effects of a drug.

Anti-inflammatory Remedies

These drugs are often used to help reduce pain and are commonly called Non-Steroidal Anti-Inflammatory Drugs (NSAIDs). Over-the-counter (OTC) NSAIDs include aspirin and ibuprofen (Advil®, Motrin®). Prescription NSAIDs in Canada include naproxen (Naprosyn®) and celecoxib (Celebrex®). These drugs have been around for a relatively long time but, in fact, have been around a very short time compared to some herbal remedies.

Anti-inflammatory herbs can reduce pain by decreasing the inflammation. Inflammation of a tissue subsequent to injury or disease can be entirely or partially responsible for the pain. The mechanism of action of NSAIDs is the inhibition of prostaglandins. Prostaglandins are involved in inflammation and pain. Some NSAIDs also have a non-prostaglandin mechanism of action that contributes to its effectiveness. Sometimes you read about drugs that are COX inhibitors. COX is the abbreviation for cyclooxygenase and this enzyme system is involved in the production of prostaglandins. COX-1 and COX-2 inhibitors are, therefore, drugs that act via the prostaglandin mechanism of action.

NSAIDs can be effective in relieving inflammation and pain due to muscle ache, menstrual pain, headache, low back pain, arthritis,

Over the short term, these drugs alone may provide sufficient pain relief, but the pain will return if the condition is not treated. Many times an anti-inflammatory drug is not sufficient to overcome the pain. The physician may have to use other drugs, such as analgesics and muscle relaxants, or turn to unconventional drugs like antidepressants for pain relief.

When used at the recommended dosages and dose frequency, these anti-inflammatory drugs can be effective pain killing medications. Over-dose or long term use can result in toxicity to the body, such as gastrointestinal injury (e.g. dyspepsia, peptic ulcers, bleeding), renal toxicity (e.g. acute renal failure, nephritic syndrome, worsening of hypertension), cardiovascular effects (antiplatelet properties of aspirin, coronary risk) and hepatic injury. These pharmaceutical agents are known to cause toxicity even when used at the recommended dosages. Some people are more susceptible than others. Sometimes it is the combination of drugs taken in a day that can lead to an interaction and ultimately toxicity.

Drug Quality

We tend to only worry about the quality of natural health products, but if we look at the news releases over the last two years, we will perhaps be surprised to see the number of pain killer over-the-counter (OTC) medications recalled from the market. These recalls were associated with the quality of the products. The issue included contamination of the products during manufacturing by other ingredients. Be vigilant when buying OTC pain killers and visit Health Canada's website that lists recalled drugs:
1. Visit the media room at Health Canada for the latest advisories and recalls at http://www.hc-sc.gc.ca/ahc-asc/media/advisories-avis/index-eng.php
2. Visit the drug recall listing at Health Canada: http://www.hc-sc.gc.ca/dhp-mps/compli-conform/recall-retrait/_list/index-eng.php

Analgesic Remedies

When we hear of analgesics we either think of Tylenol® or narcotic drugs like Dilaudid®. Some people also think of Motrin® as an analgesic. From a pain relief point of view, both are correct since analgesia is defined as the reduction or elimination of pain. From a pharmacological point of view (e.g. mechanism of action on the body to reduce pain), the term analgesic is used to define ingredients that act on a target within the body. Its action is what gives us the feeling that the pain is reduced. In other words, the ingredient blocks or stops the signal of pain to the brain which usually interprets this signal to tell us that it hurts.

Some of the pharmaceutical ingredients relieve pain not by acting at the site of the body's injury but by acting directly on our brain that interprets this hurt signal. Other pharmaceutical ingredients act directly at the site and stop the signal from going to the brain.

Acetaminophen (e.g. Tylenol®) has been around since the early 1950s and remains a very good first choice analgesic. Patients should never take more than 4 grams per day of acetaminophen. Acetaminophen is found in both OTC and prescription pain medications. Compared to many other analgesics, acetaminophen has a very good safety profile in terms of undesirable side effects. Its most common side effect is nausea. Acetaminophen may cause liver toxicity when overdoses are taken and, when taken chronically, it can cause liver damage.

The United States Food and Drug Administration (FDA) has asked manufacturers of acetaminophen prescription products (e.g. acetaminophen + hydrocodone (Lortab®) and oxycodone + acetaminophen (Percocet®)) to reduce the strength of tablets and capsules to 325 mg per pill. Additional information on this issue is available at: http://www.fda.gov/Drugs/DrugSafety/ucm239821.htm. In addition, the FDA is forcing manufacturers to add a black box warning to the label of all prescription products containing acetaminophen stating that there is a potential for severe liver injury, and allergic reactions (e.g. swelling of the face, mouth, and throat, difficulty breathing, itching, or rash). This change is not required for OTC acetaminophen products, since these warnings already appear on the label.

Unfortunately, many pharmaceutical drugs that act as analgesics have undesirable side effects and many also cause physical dependence. Both of these properties severely limit the physician's ability to relieve pain while maintaining the patient's quality of life. Many of us have taken narcotics and remember waking up the next morning with hangover-like symptoms. This is just one of the side effects experienced by people taking opioid narcotics. Opioid narcotics are ingredients that act on opioid receptors in our body and their action on the receptor results in blocking the signal of pain. The other side effects of opioid narcotics range from abnormal dreams, agitation, aggression, apprehension, attention disturbances, impaired coordination, depression, confusion, cognitive disorder, dizziness, drowsiness, dysphoria, euphoria, hallucinations, headache, insomnia, physical dependence, memory impairment, mood alterations, nervousness, panic attacks, etc. A full list of these is available from your pharmacist.

Although the thought of having the above side effects sounds negative, it is important to remember that they do provide pain relief in situations where no other agents are able to help the patient, especially in cases where the pain is unbearable to the patient. When agents have important side effects, it is even more important to adhere to the recommendations made by the physician and or pharmacist. Talk to your physician or pharmacist about any other drugs, or natural health products, that you are taking, as these could be factors that make you susceptible to getting some of these side effects. Some natural health products, such as herbs, can also be a factor that makes you more vulnerable to the effects of a drug.

To some people it is surprising to hear that antidepressant medications are used as analgesics. In fact, some of these drugs have been used for many years to relieve pain in specific conditions like fibromyalgia, migraines, and neuropathies from diabetes. Some of the better antidepressants used include tricyclic antidepressants (TCAs) (e.g. Amitriptyline®, Desipr-amine®), serotonin-selective reuptake inhibitors commonly referred to as SSRIs (e.g. Paxil®, citalopram®), and selective serotonin and norepinephrine reuptake inhibitors (referred to as SNRIs) (*e.g.* Cymbalta®, Effexor®). Clinical studies demonstrated that these drugs can be effective analgesics at dosages lower than what is used to treat conditions like depression.

Although the efficacy of these drugs in relieving pain may be good, their side effects often lead to the patient stopping the medication. In simple terms, keep in mind that these drugs were initially designed to act on the brain to help patients recover from disorders like depression or obsessive compulsion. Simply, these drugs act on the brain's chemistry to correct the imbalances that are responsible for the disorder. Based on this primary activity of the drug, it is not surprising to find that the side effects in a person with no neurological-related disorder, like depression, are unbearable. The exact mechanism of action for the pain relief of antidepressants is not known, but it certainly is a result of the drugs action on targets within our brain or spinal cord (considered part of the central nervous system).

TCAs demonstrated good efficacy at low dosages but patients cannot tolerate the strong sedative and anticholinergic (e.g. acts on nerves to reduce spasms of smooth muscles) effects. Interestingly, the newer antidepressant medications (e.g. SSRIs and SNRIs) are considered to have fewer side effects than the TCAs. Paxil®, an SSRI, which has clinical trial evidence of pain relief, unfortunately causes intolerable side effects in many patients despite what pharmacologists thought. These side effects include anxiety, agitation, abnormal dreams, impaired concentration, depersonalization, amnesia, confusion, muscle pain, muscle twitching, muscle weakness, joint pain, etc.

In cases of severe pain, several drugs may be given to obtain more relief. Some health professionals may add an NSAID to the daily treatment with acetaminophen to further reduce pain. If the patient is still in pain, the professional may then add a weak opioid acting drug to try to reduce the pain. This pharmacological approach to pain relief should only be performed by a health-care professional, as there are many implications to combining drugs, ranging from potential drug-drug interactions to additive or synergistic effects, that can result from the combination.

Drugs that potentiate the pain relief when given in combination with an analgesic are referred to as adjuvant-analgesic drugs (e.g. Clonidine® which is an alpha-2-adrenergic agonist). They are referred to as adjuvant analgesics, and not as analgesics, because based on its mechanism of action the pharmaceutical manufacturer did not initially develop the drug for pain relief.

Lyrica® is an analgesic and was the first drug approved for the treatment of fibromyalgia. It is a prescription analgesic that is also used to treat neuropathic pain. It also has side effects that some patients find undesirable, such as dizziness, ataxia, etc. In cases of severe neuropathic pain, it may be combined with other pain killers, such as opioid narcotics.

Muscle Relaxant Drugs

The class of products called skeletal muscle relaxants (e.g. Flexeril®) is used to treat muscle spasms associated with painful musculoskeletal conditions. These drugs are often used in combination with analgesics to obtain pain relief. For example, patients with L4 or L5 disc hernias may get episodes of severe muscle cramping in their lower limbs. Flexeril® is commonly used as a muscle relaxant to treat these muscle spasms.

The undesirable side effects of Flexeril® include drowsiness, dizziness, confusion, irritability, reduced mental acuity, skeletal muscle weakness, etc.

Other Drugs

Other pharmaceutical drugs like benzodiazepines (e.g. Clonazepam®, Diazepam®) are used to help relieve pain. Benzodiazepines have been shown clinically to help some patients with fibromyalgia by relaxing tense, painful muscles along with helping the patient obtain deep sleep.

Another class of pharmaceutical drugs called alpha-2-adrenergic agonists (e.g. Clonidine®) provides pain relief by acting at three different sites: the brain, spinal cord and in peripheral tissues. This class of drugs is used for neuropathic pain.

Physicians may also resort to other types of pharmaceutical drugs when trying to manage pain. For example, physicians may prescribe calcitonin in cases where patients with osteoporosis develop bone fractures. The calcitonin will reduce the risk of fractures and act as an analgesic since its bone "repair" activities will result in pain relief.

Topical Products

The use of topical creams and gels is common to help relieve pain. These products may contain anti-inflammatory, counter-irritants or anaesthetics.

Topical capsaicin products have been used to treat persistent pain in conditions like diabetic neuropathy, osteoarthritis and rheumatoid arthritis. During the first days of application some patients may obtain a burning sensation, but it is common to become tolerant to this effect. Because the burning sensation can be quite uncomfortable, it is recommended to begin using low strength capsaicin products for several days. Once tolerant to the burning sensation you can change to a stronger level of capsaicin. Be sure to wash your hands and fingers thoroughly and avoid touching any part of your body, especially your mouth and eyes, as trace amounts of capsaicin will cause burning. Even following a thorough wash, there may be sufficient traces of capsaicin to cause burning of your mouth.

Topical products containing lidocaine, an anesthetic, can be used to relieve local pain in conditions like neuropathic pain (e.g. post herpetic neuralgia) and arthritis.

Chapter 2
USING HERBS TO TREAT PAIN

The purpose of this chapter is to provide information on the different approaches that are used to treat pain. Keep in mind that pain is, in fact, a signal that the body needs help to solve a pathophysiological disturbance, or it is simply telling us that it has just been injured. Pain can be of short duration as is the case following a traumatic physical injury (e.g. bruised muscle following sports injury), it can persist for months and years as a continuous signal of the pathophysiological problem (e.g. lower back disc hernia, osteoarthritis, solid tumour), or it can be reoccurring due to the pathophysiology of the medical condition (e.g. anxiety triggered migraines).

The practitioner has to consider two aspects of pain: firstly, reducing moderate to severe pain rapidly to help the patient have a better quality of life and often to manage the pain-induced insomnia; and secondly, there will be some degree of pain that remains as long as the medical condition is not repaired or cured. In other words, the patient may continuously experience or have a recurring milder, but chronic, pain even after the acute pain is reduced and the condition or cause is being managed. Managing these two types of pain will either involve using different remedies or different dosages of the same remedies. It is extremely important to rapidly reduce the degree of the acute pain and this, in the majority of cases, is achievable with herbal remedies. Managing chronic pain will be relatively simpler, but it will also be a longer process as pain is usually associated with an underlying condition or injury. To recover-repair, the body needs restful sleep, as well as remaining calm (e.g. anxiety reduced). Stress on its own can be responsible for some, or even be the factor that initiates the pathophysiological disorder.

The population of patients on pain medications is increasing as the Canadian population ages. These patients are looking for alternatives, since their quality of life is deteriorating because of the side effects of these medications. Herbal remedies are an under-utilized tool for the management of pain. When used appropriately, herbal remedies relieve pain in patients that choose not to use pharmaceutical drugs, or in patients that take herbs as complementary medicine to drugs. The latter allows a physician to reduce the dosages of the drugs, thus avoiding certain side effects and/or reducing the duration of treatment with narcotics or reducing the dosage of narcotics.

The narcotic medications have socio-economic consequences on the patients as these individuals can no longer effectively work due to the common effects of opioid narcotics including, but not limited to, decreased concentration ability, decreased apprehension, inhibited motor coordination, etc. Physicians are also concerned about the use of narcotics in patients due to the risk of developing physical dependence.

Herbal Pharmacology: Mimicking Pain Relief Drugs

The great majority of pharmaceutical drugs have an origin with a plant or other biological organism such as a bacterium (e.g. penicillin). Scientists study the pharmacology of active ingredients created by nature looking for new and potentially active ingredients. After identifying an active fraction of a biological material from, for example, a plant extract, they proceed to identify a single active ingredient and isolate it to study its chemical structure. It may be this ingredient that becomes the pharmaceutical drug, or the scientist may modify the chemical structure to make stronger and more potent drugs. These structure-modified molecules then become pharmaceutical drugs. Although this molecule is designed by scientists, its mother or original molecular structure came from the biological material.

The above is a very simplified overview of how pharmaceutical scientists obtain drugs from herbs. What is important to understand is that the herb extract was clinically active, and it was this known activity that led scientist to study the biological material. The known clinical use was either based on the traditional use of the herb by a shaman or from that of a specific culture. Often the pure synthetic pharmaceutical drug/molecule is several times more pharmacologically potent than the herb extract. However, pharmacological studies have shown that isolating a single ingredient from the herb usually results in toxicity (e.g. side effects); whereas, the original herb, or extract, does not cause toxicity. This concept is well accepted today. We know that toxicity does not occur with the herb or herb extract because some of the other ingredients in the plant material protect our bodies from the potential negative effects. We also recognize that the use of the herb or herb extract can actually result in superior clinical benefits. The biological material has many other ingredients that help treat the condition via the desired mechanism of action (e.g. anti-inflammatory), as well as via other modes of action (e.g. properties) that will help the patient recover, such as draining waste, trophorestorative, nervine tonic, sedative, etc. Natural practitioners can use the combination of properties of the herb or herb extract to obtain a better clinical outcome in the patient. This same approach can be used in complementary medicine.

Physicians classically combine analgesics, such as acetaminophen with Non-Steroidal Anti-Inflammatory Drugs (NSAID) to obtain non-narcotic pain relief. There are no safe and effective alternatives to acetaminophen and OTC NSAIDs. Additional pain relief is only obtained by adding a weak opioid narcotic or replacing the medications with a stronger opioid narcotic. The lack of OTC pain relief medications sometimes results in the earlier use of narcotics than what physicians desire. Managing the risk of physical dependence is a critical issue that the physician must deal with. In fact, some of the herbal remedies could become new pain relief options for the physician.

We can treat pain using herbal remedies based on a pharmacological strategy similar to how conventional medicine approaches pain management with pharmaceutical drugs. In fact, we can begin using an analgesic or anti-inflammatory herb and add additional herbs to complement the pain relief. Classically, just like physicians may begin the management of pain using Tylenol® (e.g. analgesic) and then add Motrin® (e.g. anti-inflammatory), the natural health-care practitioner can begin the therapy using herbal equivalents to these drugs. The physician will then either increase the daily dosage or begin to use minimal strength narcotics. In addition, they may decide to add muscle relaxants or use other classes of drugs (as discussed in Chapter 1 of this book).

Some natural health-care practitioners treat pain or specific medical conditions with herbal combinations that are based on traditional use, or based on naturopathic modes of action (e.g. trophorestorative nervines, toxin draining, sedative, etc.) and not on herbal pharmacology. This approach has been very successful as well.

An alternative strategy involves categorizing the herbal remedies based on their primary pharmacological properties (e.g. anti-inflammatory, analgesic, sedative, anti-spasmodic) and then approaching the management of pain from a pharmacological point of view. In others words, if an herb was a nervine tonic, had anti-inflammatory activity,

15

and drained waste, we would categorize it as an anti-inflammatory herb. Therefore, we would use this herb like we would use ibuprofen (Motrin®).

If you carefully look at the traditional use of herbs by herbalists, you will, in fact, discover that herbs tend to have been historically used in conditions where patients benefit from more than one of its pharmacological activity. A good example is **Stinging nettle** (*Urtica dioica*) and gout. This herb is both anti-inflammatory and waste draining. Gout is a form of arthritis that involves the production of uric acid, a form of metabolic waste. Deposits of uric acid are involved in the painful condition, so the elimination of the uric acid waste is critical to the therapy. This does not mean that **Stinging nettle** will not provide anti-inflammatory activity in other conditions. It only means that this herbal remedy has optimal benefits in this type of condition. Reading the Materia Medica provided in this book will help you understand how these herbs have been used for centuries to treat pain.

Simplified View of Common Treatment Strategies that Assist the Management of Pain

Cleansing/Detoxification

An important part of natural therapies involves cleansing the body prior to treating the cause of the medical condition. This strategy can also be a component of a pain relief therapy regimen.

In an ideal situation, practitioners prefer to cleanse the body of toxic waste that could directly or indirectly be responsible for the medical disorder. Once the waste is eliminated, practitioners can then focus the remedies on curing the cause of the disorder. In many cases, the pain is intense or unbearable. In such a case, the practitioner must either in parallel to the cleansing therapy, or prior to cleansing, prescribe remedies to significantly reduce the pain. In some cases, the cleansing will help reduce the pain as the toxic waste is responsible for part of the pain (e.g. gout).

The liver and kidneys, which are two of the primary emunctories, are essential for the elimination of waste. These organs may require cleansing to restore their full functional capacity for toxin elimination/draining.

There are many herbal remedies that can be used for this purpose, as well as naturopathic approaches using herbs, homeopathy, gemmotherapy, vegetables or fruits as cleansing remedies, such as purge cures, fruit cures, etc. The therapy recommended by the practitioner will depend on many factors, such as the patient's tolerance to relatively stronger intestinal purging versus a milder but longer treatment for purging. Subsequent to purging, the practitioner may decide to regenerate the organs using therapies, such as gemmotherapy.

The other primary emunctories include the gall bladder, intestines, and sweat and sebaceous glands. The secondary emunctories include the mucous membranes of the uterus, stomach and respiratory tract. Naturopathic practitioners have different therapies to optimize the elimination of toxins and metabolic waste.

Anti-inflammatory Herbal Remedies

Anti-inflammatory remedies are often required to help reduce the pain. They help reduce pain by decreasing the inflammation. Inflammation of a tissue subsequent to injury or disease can be entirely or partially responsible for the pain. Over the short term, these remedies alone may provide sufficient pain relief, but the pain will return if the condition is not treated. In other words, the pain may return if the condition that caused/causes the inflammation is not cured or adequately managed. The practitioner may have to use other remedies, like analgesics and antispasmodics, when the anti-inflammatory remedy is not sufficient to overcome the pain.

In conventional medicine, it is common to administer 2 or 3 different medications to help relieve the pain. For example, an anti-inflammatory drug may be pre-scribed along with an analgesic and/or a muscle relaxant. In the case of some drugs, the physician may increase the dose of the medication to obtain more relief. What limit the number of drugs used in combination and/or the dose escalations are the safety/toxicity and potential drug-drug interactions that may occur. In addition, adding narcotic type analgesics to the patient's treatment adds the risk of developing physical dependence (e.g. addiction).

Herbal anti-inflammatory remedies are natural alternatives to pharmaceutical pain medications like Motrin® (Ibuprofen™) or Celebrex® (Celecoxib™). Natural remedies are made from either a single herb or a blend of several herbs. The following herbs (or part of the herb) are recognized as effective anti-inflammatory remedies, and this clinical benefit is possible because of the herbs' pharmacological activity: **Black currant** (*Ribes nigrum*), **Boswellia** (*Boswellia sacra*), **Stinging nettle** (*Urtica dioica*), **Turmeric** (*Curcuma longa*), **Devil's claw** (*Harpagophytum procumbens*) and **Common Figwort** (*Scrophularia nodosa*). When given at the appropriate dosages and dose frequency, these natural anti-inflammatory herbal agents can be effective substitutes for pharmaceutical pain medications while avoiding the safety concerns of the pharmaceutical medications.

Keep in mind that herbs are safe as long as they are used according to their recommended use. In other words, taking dosages that are two or more times greater than the recommended dose could cause side effects. Side effects may occur because you would be receiving much higher levels than has been safely used historically. Also, the traditional use of herbs involves the use of the same plant species and plant part (e.g. root, bark). The safest way to ensure that you are using the correct herb is to go by the proper name of the plant. (For example, use the proper name **Scrophularia nodosa** and not the common name **Figwort**.) This also applies to the desired efficacy, because herbs that have similar common names may not have the same clinical activity. For example, **Meadow-sweet** (*Filipendula ulmaria*), which is also known as **Queen-of-the-Meadow** is an herb commonly used in Europe and Asia for treating pain. **Queen of the Meadow,** which is also known as **Gravel root,** (*Eupatorium purpureum*) is a different plant used to treat various kidney diseases.

Analgesic Herbal Remedies

Many people are surprised to discover that herb extracts can be effective analgesics. A simple example is the herb **Meadowsweet** (*Filipendula ulmaria*). The pharmaceutical drug Aspirin™ was named after *Spiraea ulmaria*, which is the old name for **Meadowsweet** (van Wyk & Wink 2010) and where Aspirin's original active ingredient was derived.

Some of the herbs with analgesic activity can be used to treat pain just like pharmaceutical drugs, such as Tylenol®. This includes combining analgesic herbs with anti-inflammatory herbs to obtain stronger pain relief. The herbs with analgesic activity discussed in this book are **Boswellia** (*Boswellia sacra or serrata*), **California poppy** (*Eschscholzia californica*), **Common Figwort** (*Scrophularia nodosa*), **Corydalis** (*Corydalis yanhusuo*), **Devil's claw** (*Harpagophytum procumbens*), **White peony** (*Paeonia lactiflora*) and **White willow** (*Salix alba*). These herbal analgesics pharmacologically work via mechanisms of action that are identical to those used by pharmaceutical analgesic drugs. Some of the pharmacological analgesic modes of action include activity on the opioid and serotonin receptors, as well as others.

Plants such as **California poppy** (*Eschscholzia californica*) are unique in that they provide analgesia via the opioid and serotonin receptors. This pharmacological activity is highly interesting, as it has recently been demonstrated that the combination of molecules that act on opioid and serotonin receptors results in synergistic pain relief. This herbal agent is also unique in that it not only acts as an analgesic; it also is a hypnotic and mild sedative. It is recognized as non-narcotic because it does not induce physical dependence. These properties make the herbal agent optimal for management of pain-related insomnia. In fact, preclinical research shows that this plant acts on opioid, serotonin and norepinephrine systems for pain relief, making it an ideal alternative to the use of antidepressants in the treatment of pain. This is especially true for patients that do not tolerate antidepressants.

Physicians commonly prescribe antidepressants for the management of pain and pain-associated insomnia in patients with fibromyalgia and diabetic neuropathy. The antidepressants are used because these drugs increase the serotonin levels in the Central Nervous System (CNS), as well as acting on the norepinephrine system. The use of anti-depressants is growing in popularity subsequent to clinical trials showing their superiority over intramuscular morphine (Moore et al 2003).

In cases of severe pain, several analgesic drugs may be given in combination to obtain more relief. Some refer to these additional drugs as adjuvant-analgesic drugs (e.g. Clonidine® which is an alpha-2-adrenergic agonist), since they potentiate the pain relief when given in combination with an analgesic. They are referred to as adjuvant analgesics because, based on their mechanism of action, the pharmaceutical manufacturer did not initially develop the drug for pain relief. In a sense, herbs have a similar adjuvant property, in that you obtain additional pain relief via the other pharmacological activities of the herb, such as its antispasmodic or visceral relaxant activity.

Antispasmodic and Relaxant Remedies

Muscle spasms commonly occur in patients with moderate-to-severe lower back pain associated with irritation of the spinal roots by herniated discs. The 'antispasmodic' drug of choice for physicians is Flexeril®, which is a neuromuscular blocking agent. A natural alternative is **Scullcap** (*Scutellaria lateriflora*). **Scullcap** is well known for its antispasmodic properties and its calming and anxiolytic properties. The patient benefits from both sets of properties.

Counter-irritant Remedies

Some of the effective topical gels for local pain relief contain ingredients called counterirritants. The following are examples of counterirritant ingredients: **Menthol, camphor, eucalyptus oil, thymol,** and **clove oil**. These latter types of agents relieve pain by reducing the inflammation of deep structures via their topical effect on the skin. This mechanism of action results in a cooling and/or heating sensation on the surface of the skin. When the products are adequately formulated, the patient will experience the sensation that the ingredients are penetrating deeply into the tissue.

Using a product that is adequately formulated is important because skin irritation can occur when the level of these ingredients is too high in the formulation. In Canada, one way to ensure that a product is safe is to look for the Natural Products Number (NPN) on the label. The NPN number is the only way for a consumer to know that a product was evaluated by Health Canada, and that the government regulators determined that it is both safe and effective.

Regeneration-Repair

In many cases, part of the cure will require that the practitioner regenerate or repair the tissue. For example, a critical aspect to reducing and preventing pain in osteoarthritis is helping the body regenerate the cartilage tissue in a joint. Pain in osteoarthritis is frequently associated with the loss of cartilage from the degeneration.

There are some well-established therapies that can be used by the practitioner to regenerate tissue, such as gemmotherapy. These therapies involve the use of diluted extracts prepared from the bud or other immature parts of a plant. This therapy was inspired by the science of homeopathic drainage, and the concentration of the extract falls somewhere between those used by herbalists (e.g. phytotherapy) and those used by homeopathic practitioners.

A very difficult pain condition is osteoarthritis of the knee. It is simple to understand why this condition is painful. Just picture the weight of your body on the knee joint and that the joint is like a ball in a casing covering part of its surface. When the joint is healthy, the ball has a cushion protecting it from the friction that occurs as it rotates within the casing. In the case of osteoarthritis, the cushion has begun to shrink and eventually the entire cushion is lost. When a major part of the cushion is lost, the ball rotates within the casing but now the two surfaces rub, which creates friction and the body translates this into pain. The heavier we are, the more pressure there will be on the joint.

Part of the therapy must involve reducing or preventing this cushion from degenerating and, depending on multiple factors, help regenerate this cushion. These therapies involve administering remedies over a long term to the patient. Initially, these remedies help reduce the pain by reducing the degeneration of the cushion. Over time they help the body's vital energies rebuild or regenerate the cushion. From a pathophysiological point of view, the degenerative process is in fact quite complex, and success requires that the therapy reduce or stop the inflammatory process that is directly or indirectly responsible for the degeneration of the cushion. The therapeutic agents prescribed must not only stop the inflammatory process that involves cells of our body programmed to start and maintain the inflammation, but also prevent the cells of the cushion from being destroyed by the inflammatory process. It is also complex in that the therapies must stop cells that cause the harm but, at the same time, protect other cells that the body/cushion requires. A challenge that is extremely complex from a pharmaceutical drug point of view, but certainly not impossible, for natural remedies that help the vital forces of the body tackle this challenge.

There are many studies that have demonstrated that the above is achievable using blends of herbal remedies along with chondroprotective ingredients (e.g. glucosamine sulphate, MSM, chondroitin sulphate). This research also demonstrated that what is important is avoiding ingredients that may do the opposite of what is required. For example, some ingredients may help stimulate the inflammatory cells responsible for the degeneration.

Weight Loss, Nutrition and Physical Activity

The last thing we want to hear when we are in pain is to make changes to our life style and lose weight. This is understandable because a good part of our body's energy is being used to resist the feeling of pain. The fact that body weight (e.g. obesity), poor nutrition and/or a sedentary life style possibly are playing a factor in the condition that is causing the pain is why the practitioner is going to focus part of the therapy on these. It is also why it is critical for the practitioner to rapidly reduce the acute pain level. Once the pain becomes tolerable, the patient becomes more receptive to beginning a journey into modifying their eating habits and increasing their physical activity.

Physical activity is a key component to losing weight and to the body's strength-endurance to resist disease and/or rebuild strength to a tissue following a sports injury. Numerous studies have demonstrated the effect of exercise on the immune system, and even on the ability of the brain to generate endorphins that help reduce pain.

When our body is facing conditions associated with degeneration, it is important to address the potential factors that are contributing to the degeneration, and find ways to stop the process (or at least provide the body with the elements it needs to resist). Degeneration is a natural phenomenon that our body faces as we age. Exercise and nutrition can help delay or reduce the degree of degeneration. Numerous foods contain antioxidants. Supplements or foods that contain high levels of antioxidants can be taken to help the body manage the degeneration process.

Taking only supplements for losing weight provides only short-term success in terms of duration of the weight loss, as well as the number of pounds lost. Supplements plus calorie intake reduction provide a more successful outcome to weight loss. Many successful professional weight loss programs involve calorie reduction along with increased physical activity. Key to the success of these programs is taking the person from a sedentary state to a much more active physical state, and this can be as simple as walking 30 minutes a day 3 days a week. The more intense the activity (such as a rapid walking pace) the greater will be the calorie burn. In parallel to the fat burning, the body rebuilds its muscle mass and sometimes we even feel that it is adding muscle mass to parts of our body that we never used. The ability to lose significant weight and then maintain the weight loss involves maintaining the new acquired level of physical activity, as well as learning to eat wisely. Eating wisely is as simple as following Canada's food guide (http://www.hc-sc.gc.ca/fn-an/food-guide-aliment/index-eng.php). This book is about managing pain, but do not forget the impact on our health of poor eating and the relationships between various diseases like diabetes, heart disease and cancer and nutrition. The challenge of modifying our life style is not insignificant, and muscle fatigue and cramps rapidly become obstacles to this goal. Like with many life style changes, persistence early on is important to allow these changes to become routine.

Quality of Herbal Remedies

Quality of the product is an important point to remember when buying herbal remedies, since the dosage is critical to obtaining pain relief, especially in the case of acute pain. Keep in mind the importance of using the right plant species and plant part. There have been cases of companies adulterating the product with other herbs.

Talk to your pharmacist or practitioner about the different suppliers of herbal remedies, if you are not familiar with the product brand.

Chapter 3
HERBAL COMBINATIONS

Several herbs have been used to treat pain for centuries. The combinations of herbs were based on historical use by herbalists developed over time from trial and error. Basically, herbalists learned from experience which herbs and herb parts, acted additively or synergistically to provide a stronger clinical response.

Some herbalists add herbs to a remedy to help protect the stomach from irritation, protect the liver from toxins, and/or help the kidneys eliminate waste. Other practitioners may cleanse the body before giving the herbal treatment, then again after the patient's therapy. These latter practices will depend on the health condition, the duration of treatment, the patient's health and lifestyle (e.g. diet), and the practitioner's clinical experience. Today scientific studies have shown that some of the herbs added for protective reasons also directly contribute to treating the condition; for example, Turmeric (*Curcuma longa*) and inflammation. Turmeric is recognized for its anti-inflammatory properties, as well as its liver protective benefits.

Some companies perform experimental studies using cell cultures of healthy and/or sick human tissues to try to elucidate the additive or synergistic relationships between herbs. This research can go as far as studying the chemokine and cytokine levels or their gene expressions.

This research can help narrow down what combinations work effectively together. But, in the end, good old clinical evidence will be the final judge. This experimental approach was used by a Canadian natural health innovative company to try to understand the synergistic relationship between the herbal ingredients contained in its anti-inflammatory formulation. However, the formulation itself was based on the clinical experience of herbalists. The company successfully demonstrated the additive effects between some herbs, and also demonstrated synergistic effects between other herbs, using classical pharmacological animal models. The models used were the same ones used by major pharmaceutical companies.

The company's herbal formulation included herbs for their ant-inflammatory activity, liver and stomach protection and waste elimination by the kidney. The company also demonstrated using pharmaceutical animal models that they could reduce the progression of osteoarthritis and even help regenerate the cartilage tissue.

The above company's research activities allowed the scientists to elucidate the mechanism of action of the herbal blend. Ultimately they clearly demonstrated the power of good herbal formulations based on sound herbal and natural medicine sciences.

Different herbal therapeutic approaches have been used over the centuries ranging from that of the Doctrine of Signatures, Eclectic physicians, to that of low dose approaches. Some of these approaches are based on using low dosages of herbs relative to dosages considered pharmacologically active. Don't mistake my comment to mean that it is not clinically effective! In fact, many health conditions are effectively treated using a low dosage therapeutic approach.

Rapid reduction of pain requires a very different approach. Keep in mind that there is a subjective factor in the degree that you feel pain. Basically, some people may describe the same degree and type of pain as being bearable and others may find it so intolerable that their daily activities and sleep are disturbed. A reduction in the level of pain by at least 50% may give you a tolerable level of pain but other people may require over 80% reduction to feel comfortable. To rapidly reduce pain the body requires relatively high dosages of the herbs.

The high dosages are required to rapidly block the pain receptors in the body and/or to inhibit the inflammation pathways to reduce the swelling which may itself be fully or partially responsible for feeling severe pain. Partial blocking or partial inhibition of inflammatory pathways may work well in chronic diseases and/or non-pain conditions. But when you are in moderate or severe pain it hurts, and you need to suppress the pain as fast as possible. Even people with mild pain may, over time, find it unbearable or that it affects their daily activities or sleep.

In conventional medicine, the rapid pain reduction would be achieved by giving analgesic and anti-inflammatory drugs, and, in some cases, it would include giving an antispasmodic drug. Over the centuries, pharmaceutical and conventional medical sciences developed drugs that are pure molecules. These pure molecules can be very strong blockers of a receptor (a structure in our bodies where molecules bind to it to block or induce a biological response) or inflammation pathway. Years of clinical studies and conventional medical practice demonstrated that some types of pains are effectively treated using only an analgesic drug (e.g. acetaminophen or hydromorphone) or anti-inflammatory drug (e.g. Ibuprofen or Celebrex®). More severe conditions may require giving both analgesic and anti-inflammatory drugs in combination. In some cases, the patient may need to add an antispasmodic or muscle relaxant drug to further ease the pain. A muscle spasm or muscle cramp can be responsible for the pain or discomfort preventing daily activities and sleep.

With three main categories of drugs, conventional medical doctors can effectively manage the majority of pain conditions. These three categories are analgesic, anti-inflammatory (NSAID) and muscle relaxant.

In the case of analgesics, conventional medicine has several choices ranging from a non-narcotic, like acetaminophen, to narcotics like hydromorphone and morphine. Over the last years, the SSRIs and SNRIs have become popular treatment choices for fibromyalgia and other chronic pain conditions like diabetic neuropathy. Other drugs, like Lyrica that act on different systems in the central nervous system (e.g. GABA), are also effective analgesics. The negative side of many of these medications is their "pureness" or the fact that they strongly block a pathway. Side effects that can be unbearable or unacceptable for the patient often push the patient to look for alternative remedies. Some of these side effects are due to the very strong binding or blocking action of the drug. Herbal remedies are different in that the formulation contains hundreds of molecules, and the so called known medicinal molecules of the herb act on multiple systems in our body. Clinically, the herbs, when used at an adequate dosage, will provide just as effective pain relief, but through their actions on multiple systems (e.g. acting on both opioid and serotonin receptor systems in our central nervous system). In general, the herbal remedies are recognized as having few side effects, if any. But side effects are a question of product quality, dosage, duration of use, and potential drug-herb interactions. As a general rule, there will be far fewer side effects with a natural remedy when it is as per the recommended directions of use.

Since herbal remedies have few side effects compared to the synthetic drugs, herbalists can use relatively higher dosages of the herb to rapidly suppress the pain. As the pain decreases, the level of the herbal product can be adjusted.

Conventional medicine will treat insomnia by prescribing drugs from the pharmacological class of benzodiazepines, SNRI or SSRI. Many patients do not like taking these drugs because of their side effects, including those that have residual side effects the next morning (e.g. agitation, reduced ability to concentrate, etc). When taken daily for several months, it is not easy to stop the medication, as some people experience withdrawal types of side effects.

Herbal Combinations that Mimic Conventional Drugs

One approach to reducing moderate or severe pain is to use herbs according to their pharmacological properties; that is mimicking the mode of action of conventional pharmaceutical drugs. This is easily done by using herbs according to their pharmacological classification described in Table 1 (page 38), and making formulations by combining analgesic, anti-inflammatory and antispasmodic herbs together. The primary goal (Step #1) is reducing the severe pain very rapidly. Therefore, the use of herbs should be based on mimicking the conventional drugs; in other words, use of analgesic and anti-inflammatory herbs. Once the pain is controlled (Step #2) the treatment strategy (e.g. choice of herbs) should be modified to focus on the condition and/or chronic pain. Some of the herbs initially used to rapidly reduce the pain should be kept for managing pain flare ups. This second stage of treatment needs to consider condition-specific herbs.

In some cases, the herbs have more than one property and therefore the herb itself may act as both an analgesic and anti-inflammatory agent (e.g. Devil's claw (*Harpagophytum procumbens*)). In other cases, the herb may have a well-established historical use in a specific pain condition (e.g. Black cohosh (*Cimicifuga racemosa*), Stinging nettle). Some herbs will also have sedative properties and these can be used at night to not only relieve pain but also to help you fall asleep. These herbs have dual action: pain suppression plus sedation to sleep.

When taking herbs that sedate, be careful if you are to drive a car or perform any potential hazardous task as they can cause drowsiness. Do not underestimate the clinical potential of some herbs because, when used at appropriate dosages, they can be quite potent.

In cases of mild-to-moderate pain, a single herb that is both analgesic and anti-inflammatory (referred to as Non-Steroidal Anti-Inflammatory Drug or NSAID in the table) may be sufficient to relieve the pain within 24 to 48 hours. Moderate-to-severe pain will require relatively higher dosages and may also require the use of an antispasmodic herb. The relief should begin within the first 48 hours but may take several days to obtain optimal benefit. When pain keeps you awake at night, include an herb that also has sedative properties.

History has demonstrated through traditional use that some herbs have very specific efficacy (e.g. condition-specific herbs). Sometimes there is no pharmacological mechanistic evidence to support the observed clinical benefit in patients. These condition-specific herbs should always be considered for this medical condition, mainly because of their recognized benefit over centuries. Be sure to verify that there are no safety reasons why you should not be taking the herb and, when in doubt, talk to a health-care practitioner or pharmacist. For example, Black cohosh (*Cimicifuga racemosa*) is a condition-specific herb for the relief of muscle and joint pain associated with rheumatic conditions and neuralgia (e.g. sciatica). Rheumatic conditions include rheumatoid arthritis, osteoarthritis, and fibrositis. If you had rheumatoid arthritis, you would want to include Black cohosh (*Cimicifuga racemosa*) in the herbal ingredients. A simple combination of Black cohosh (*Cimicifuga racemosa*) with Common Figwort (*Scrophularia nodosa*) would provide analgesia, as well as anti-inflammatory activity, as well as the benefits of a condition-specific herb. This combination has been shown to be effective in patients with mild-to-moderate arthritis (e.g. swollen finger or knee joints). It may happen once in a while that you perform more strenuous activities and this can lead to pain flare ups. These flare ups can involve severe pain and stop you from falling or staying asleep. When this happens, the use of a topical gel with counter-irritants can be used during the day or before bedtime to locally reduce the pain. Alternatively, you can add a supplement containing California poppy (*Eschscholzia californica*) to provide additional analgesia and mild sedative activity to help you sleep. When the more severe pain is persistent, you should consult a health-care practitioner to either adjust the dosages of the herbs you are taking, add new herbal remedies, or modify the entire treatment plan. It is important to consult to avoid over-dosing and to exclude the possibility of a new medical condition that is responsible for this increased pain. Remember that pain is a signal to the body that something is wrong, and a sudden or gradual increase in pain may not be caused by the existing/known condition, but by a different and new disease.

Another example of an ideal formulation is the simple combination of Black cohosh (*Cimicifuga racemosa*) with Stinging nettle for gout, a rheumatic condition. Black cohosh is the condition-specific herb and Stinging nettle is an anti-inflammatory herb with activity associated with the elimination of uric acid from the body. Uric acid is an important metabolic waste associated with painful gout. Keep in mind that we are talking about relieving pain associated with the condition and not curing the condition. Relieving the pain is an essential part of healing and, once suppressed, the practitioner can then focus on curing the disease, which may take time.

An optimal formulation for menstrual pain is the simple combination of Black cohosh (*Cimicifuga racemosa*) with Scullcap (*Scutellaria lateriflora*). Scullcap has been shown to relieve the pain associated with menstruation. This benefit has been associated to its antispasmodic activity. Other than Black cohosh's benefits in relieving menstrual pain, it has been traditionally used to help relieve premenstrual pain and to help relieve symptoms associated with menopause. If you get menstrual pains regularly, you should begin taking these types of products a few days before the day of the menstrual cycle that they normally occur. This will help prevent the occurrence and/or severity. It may happen one month that the pain is more severe. On those days, the use of herbs like California poppy (*Eschscholzia californica*) at night can help reduce the pain and provide sedative activity to help you sleep. Anti-inflammatory remedies may also help reduce more severe episodes of menstrual pain.

Some herbs like Devil's claw (*Harpagophytum procumbens*) have had numerous clinical trials demonstrate its pain relief benefits in lower back pain (e.g. disc hernia), osteoarthritis and rheumatoid arthritis. These trials demonstrated its strength as an anti-inflammatory agent, therefore it should be part of a general anti-inflammatory formulation. Some products combine Devil's claw with other anti-inflammatory herbs, and/or omega-3 fatty acids, that target different inflammation pathways to try to obtain a more efficacious response. Some of these combination products have been shown to be quite good anti-inflammatory remedies for pain relief. Some researchers believe that a blend of relatively lower dosages of several herbs, that target a different inflammation pathway, will provide an additive or synergistic clinical benefit. Clinical studies performed by health-care practitioners have confirmed that some of these blends can be effective.

California poppy (*Eschscholzia californica*) is an optimal herb for pain management because of its dual activities. It is a strong analgesic with sedative properties, and this can be used to maximize relief when night pain prevents you from sleeping. Studies on the pain relief mechanism of action of California poppy and its isoquinoline alkaloids demonstrated that its analgesic effect is mainly through the opioid systems and other systems such as the serotonin receptors (e.g. receptors involved in pain, anxiety, sedation, etc.). Only a partial role has been associated to an adrenergic mechanism. Isoquinoline alkaloids are considered by pharmacologists as the active components of the herb, and these alkaloids are molecules that are like derivatives of codeine and morphine. Experimental studies performed using a concentrated extract of California poppy (*Eschscholzia californica*) confirmed its sedative, anxiolytic and analgesic effects.

Studies in humans have shown that the sedative and analgesic effects are dependent on the dosage. At lower dose levels, the analgesic activity of California poppy (*Eschscholzia californica*) can be maximized in combination with an anti-inflammatory agent such as Devil's claw (*Harpagophytum procumbens*). This type of combination makes a good remedy for relieving pain during the day while avoiding potential drowsiness.

At relatively higher dose levels of California poppy, the product will be sufficiently strong to relieve pain alone as an analgesic. At these relatively higher dose levels, the drowsiness will become an issue for people that drive cars or are involved in jobs that require complete attention due to potential dangers, such as those involved with heavy machinery. There is an individual aspect to the effect of California poppy on drowsiness, in that some people may experience strong sedation the first time they take the herb, and others may simple not experience any drowsiness. The drowsiness will obviously be more pronounced on days when you are already tired.

When taking California poppy on a daily basis, with time, some people will experience less drowsiness. However, its effect in keeping you in a deep and restful sleep remains despite the effect on drowsiness. Herbal medical practice and clinical studies have shown that California poppy can effectively be used to manage insomnia because of its effects in inducing a deep and restful sleep. In fact, restful sleep is a critical part of allowing the body to recover from disease. People with fibromyalgia have found California poppy to be quite beneficial when taken twice a day, and it has helped them with both their pain and insomnia. People with this condition should speak to their health practitioner about California poppy and see if it can potentially help them.

As with any herb or pharmaceutical product, some people can have experiences that are opposite to that of the majority. Some of the prescription sleep aids are known to keep some patients awake at night (e.g. cause insomnia). California poppy can also have the opposite effect and cause insomnia in a small percentage of people.

Studies in humans have also shown an effect on dreams that is dependent on the dose of California poppy (*Eschscholzia californica*). This is not surprising, since herbalists have traditionally used tinctures of California poppy to treat nightmares. A very small number of people taking relatively low doses of California poppy will observe that it induces pleasant dreams. These are not hallucinations! As the dose level of the herb is increased, the percentage of people that observe a pleasant effect on dreams increases. From a pharmacological point of view, this is not surprising, since drugs that act on serotonin receptors are known to affect dreams.

California poppy (*Eschscholzia californica*) is a powerful herb for managing pain and sleep. Talk to your health-care practitioner about it and, especially about what dose level is right for you. Remember that some people will have drowsiness, and taking it during the day may not be right for you. If you are looking for an effective sleep aid product, especially when pain keeps you up at night, look for products that contain combinations of California poppy with tranquilizing or sedative herbs, such as: Hops (*Humulus lupulus*), Scullcap (*Scutellaria lateriflora*), Passionflower (*Passiflora incarnata*), Lemon Balm (*Melissa officinalis*), and/or Valerian (*Valeriana officinalis*). A combination of California poppy with at least one of these makes a very good sleep aid.

The use of herbs in combination with pharmaceutical drugs is discussed in Chapter 4 on

Complementary Medicine. Note that it is very important to discuss the use of California poppy (*Eschscholzia californica*) with a health professional when taking other medications for pain and or insomnia. Remember that California poppy will have additive effects with other pain and sleep medications including antidepressants and antipsychotics commonly used for managing insomnia.

OVERVIEW OF TREATMENT STRATEGY

Step #1: Focus is on rapidly reducing pain.

Step #2: Focus is on condition and treating pain flare ups.

EXAMPLE A: PAINFUL RHEUMATOID ARTHRITIS

Step #1: Use of California poppy (*Eschscholzia californica*) + Devil's claw (*Harpagophytum procumbens*) to rapidly reduce pain.

Step #2A: Use of Black cohosh (*Cimicifuga racemosa*) and Common Figwort (*Scrophularia nodosa*) to reduce inflammation and pain associated with rheumatic condition.

Step #2B: Use of California poppy (*Eschscholzia californica*) + Devil's claw (*Harpagophytum procumbens*) to reduce pain flare ups.

EXAMPLE B: LOWER BACK PAIN + INSOMNIA DUE TO PAIN

Step #1A: Use of California poppy (*Eschscholzia californica*) + Devil's claw (*Harpagophytum procumbens*) to rapidly reduce pain.

Step #1B: Use of sedative herbs to help sleep at night.

Step #1C: Addition of Scullcap (*Scutellaria lateriflora*) to reduce muscle spasms.

Step #2A: Use of a blend of anti-inflammatory herbs to reduce inflammation.

Step #2B: Use of California poppy (*Eschscholzia californica*) + HOPS to for insomnia.

EXAMPLE C: PAIN FROM SPORTS INJURY

Step #1A: Use Devil's claw (*Harpagophytum procumbens*) to rapidly reduce pain.

Step #1B: Use of California poppy (*Eschscholzia californica*) to help sleep at night.

Step #2A: Use of a blend of anti-inflammatory herbs to reduce inflammation.

Note: Use of mechanical support for injured limb and/or physiotherapy, etc.

EXAMPLE D: SEVERE PAIN ONSET

Step #1A: Use of California poppy (*Eschscholzia californica*) + Devil's claw (*Harpagophytum procumbens*) to rapidly reduce pain.

Step #1B: Use of sedative herbs to help sleep at night.

Note: Need to consult health practitioner as pain is a warning signal that something happened to your body. Even if the pain is now gone, it is important to consult as it occurred for a reason!

PRECAUTION

It is important to reduce pain but never forget that pain is a signal that something is wrong. Do not neglect consulting a health-care practitioner.

Table 1: Pharmacological Classification of herbs

Herb	Classification	
	Pain	**Other**
Black cohosh (*Cimicifuga racemosa*)	Analgesic Condition-specific for rheumatic conditions and neuralgia	Endocrine-like
Black currant (Ribes nigrum)	NSAID	
Boswellia (Boswellia sacra or Boswellia serrate)	Analgesic NSAID	Antitumor
Burdock (Arctium lappa)	Analgesic	Diuretic[1]; Depurative/ Cleansing[2]
California poppy (*Eschscholzia californica*)	Analgesic (Non-addictive) Sedative/ hypnotic	Anxiolytic
Common Figwort (*Scrophularia nodosa*)	Analgesic NSAID	Diuretic[1]; Cleansing[2]
Corydalis (*Corydalis yanhusuo*)	Analgesic Sedative	Antiarrhythmic
Devil's claw (*Harpagophytum procumbens*)	Analgesic NSAID Antirheumatic	Bitter tonic
Feverfew (Chrysanthemum parthenium)	Migraine prevention	Anti-allergic Emmena-gogue Anthelmintic

Horsetail (Equisetum arvense)	NSAID	Diuretic[1] Astringent Styptic Anti-haemorrhagic
Licorice (liquorice) (Glycyrrhiza glabra)	Antispasmodic	Muco-protective Adrenal tonic Expectorant Demulcent Mild laxative Anticariogenic Antitussive
Meadowsweet (*Filipendula ulmaria*)	Analgesic NSAID	Antacid Urinary antiseptic Muco-protective
Skullcap (*Scutellaria lateriflora*)	Antispasmodic Calmative / anti-anxiety	Nervine tonic
Stinging nettle (*Urtica dioica*) (Leaf only)	NSAID Antirheumatic	Drain uric acid waste in gout Anti-allergic Styptic (haemostatic)
Turmeric (Curcuma longa)	NSAID	Protective[3] Antiplatelet; Antioxidant; Hypo-lipidaemic; Choleretic
Valerian (*Valeriana officinalis*)	Antispasmodic Sedative	Anxiolytic;

White peony (Paeonia lactiflora)	Analgesic NSAID Antispasmodic	Cognition enhancer; Anti-allergic; Estrogen modulating
White willow (Salix alba)	Analgesic NSAID	Antipyretic

1. Increase excretion by kidneys.

2. Traditionally used in Herbal Medicine as an alterative (blood purifying properties) to help remove accumulated waste products via the kidneys, skin and mucus membranes.

3. Liver protection.

Chapter 4
COMPLEMENTARY MEDICINE

The term alternative medicine is widely used when natural remedies, like herbs, are used instead of conventional pharmaceutical drugs. For some people, this is part of their lifestyle and personal convictions. Complementary medicine is not as well known, but it involves the combination of pharmaceutical drugs and herbs (or natural remedies). When optimally combined, herbs can complement the efficacy of conventional drugs. The herbs can also be integrated with the goal of reducing the dosage level of a pharmaceutical drug as part of an approach to reduce side effects that are not well tolerated by the patient. I hope this book will encourage those of you that want a complementary medicine approach to speak to your physician about how herbs can help reduce pain, as well as treat pain-related insomnia.

In some medical conditions, complementary medicine has been used successfully. Rheumatologists are some of the first medical professionals that integrated the use of natural remedies into treatment protocols for the management of osteoarthritis. Complementary medicine will become more and more important in chronic medical conditions.

Over the last year, we have seen the desire of physicians treating pain to integrate herbal-based remedies into their medical practices. Other than efficacy, the first issues that need to be addressed are quality and safety. Quality obviously impacts safety and efficacy, because poor quality means safety concerns, as well as lack of efficacy.

Demonstrating that an herb can effectively manage pain is one challenge when dealing with physicians; but how do you integrate the herb with pain relieving drugs? Is there the potential for drug-herb interactions that put the patient at risk? Will the herb modify the metabolism of some of the drugs, thereby either reducing the efficacy or increasing the blood levels of the drug? Will the herb and the drug act on the same physiological targets within our bodies, and will this lead to an additive response? Will the herb counter the beneficial effects of the drug? There are many issues to consider, but it is doable when a company wants to enter into the complementary medicine market. The effects of some herbs are well established through well-designed clinical trials, and sufficient information is available to safely administer the herb in combination with a drug while remaining cautious.

In the case of pain management, physicians are used to treating with multiple drugs in order to reduce pain. They commonly add drugs to a prescription attempting to reduce the intolerable pain. They also try to avoid the use of narcotic drugs that have the potential of addiction (e.g. developing physical dependence).

The reason why herbs have not become an integrated part of conventional pain management has been the lack of quality products as well as the lack of scientific data. Over the years, some companies have com-mercialized low-quality products and used direct-to-consumer television ads to promote ineffective products. In some cases, the products were simply deficient in the active ingredients and, in other cases, the products were adulterated with other ingredients, such as synthetic drugs. There are well-documented cases of people dying after consuming a natural product that was adulterated with a synthetic drug. Adulteration with drugs or other ingredients is a dangerous practice, because the consumer that is sensitive or allergic to an ingredient will not be aware that he or she is about to consume a product with an ingredient that is dangerous to his or her wellbeing. Product labels need to fully disclose the ingredients in a product, so that the consumer can be consented to all ingredients that they will take.

Poor quality puts a hold on the acceptance of natural remedies by physicians. There are companies that always aimed to have high quality products and products that were both safe and efficacious. In Canada, the NPN (Natural Product Number) approval is minimal proof of quality, safety and efficacy. Health professionals still need to question companies about the quality and what scientific evidence supports the use in a specific medical condition. Natural health practitioners are becoming more and more sensitive to the same quality, safety and efficacy issues, and with time, the demand by health professionals for good products and evidence will drive out the poor quality products. Our health is important, and paying for a product that does not work is not acceptable in our society!

Do not hesitate to discuss the herbs with your physician if you believe in this approach. Many times the pain relieving drugs result in intolerable side effects. The integration of an herb into your treatment protocol may allow the physician to reduce the dose level of the drug responsible for the side effect, while preserving the desired level of efficacy.

The primary pharmacological activity of the herb, as well as any significant secondary activity, has to be taken into consideration. For example, a physician may add an analgesic herb to an analgesic drug but, usually, each of the analgesic agents will act on different pharmacological-physiological targets. Adding an analgesic herb that acts on opioid and/or serotonin receptors in the body when a patient is taking Tylenol® can be done safely. However, combining California poppy (*Eschscholzia californica*) with an SSRI or SNRI will raise safety concerns. The concerns

44

are that the herb also acts on serotonin receptors in the body, and the consequence of combining to a drug that blocks the reuptake of serotonin is not known. Just like combining an SSRI drug with an opioid agonist like hydromorphone can provide additional pain relief, combining an herb that acts on opioid receptors with an SSRI may also provide additional pain relief. Many times it is the "unknown" aspect that prevents the use of herbs in combination with drugs. Companies that sell natural remedies for the conventional medicine market have to perform research to lower these barriers and address the potential safety issues. Helping patients is not just promoting the relative safety of the herb; it is also being committed to studying the safety of the herb alone, and in combination with drugs.

Additive effects will occur when combining anti-inflammatory herbs with drug NSAIDs. Some patients do not tolerate NSAIDs (e.g. gastrointestinal irritation) or NSAIDs may be contraindicated (e.g. kidney disease). In these cases, the use of an herbal anti-inflammatory agent becomes a good pharmacological option for the physician. Of course, the physician needs to know the secondary activities of the herb (e.g. anticoagulant), as well as any potential drug-herb interactions and any known contra-indications or warnings.

Lower leg muscle cramping is common in some people with disc hernias in the lower back. Some people do not tolerate the side effects of conventional muscle relaxant drugs. In these cases, physicians can turn to herbs that have antispasmodic activity. Some herbs are even reputed for their effects in relieving lower leg muscle cramps. The pharmaceutical drug will normally specifically target muscle relaxation, but some of the herbal antispasmodics will also have additional pharmacological activities. These additional activities have to be known so that the physician can safely integrate the herb into the treatment protocol.

In my dealings with pain physicians, the discussions have always been positive irrespective of the questions and their concerns for the patient's wellbeing. In some cases, I was positively surprised to see their interest in traditional herbal medicine.

If you think about it, a physician is trained to help cure people, so it is only normal that they consider natural remedies. What has stopped physicians from using natural remedies is the uncertainty over quality, and the lack of scientific evidence on safety and efficacy of the products in treating disease.

Chapter 5
PAIN HERBAL MATERIA MEDICA

Herbs have traditionally been found to have multiple therapeutic applications. This book and its materia medica (e.g. monographs) only discuss the uses in the treatment of pain. At times, the text very briefly mentions other therapeutic applications. Therefore, for other medical conditions (e.g. non-pain) refer to another reference book to obtain the recommended doses, as well as other safety and efficacy information (such as the references Bone and van Wyk & Wink).

The monographs in this book contain detailed information on the safety of each herb, including potential interactions with drugs. To simplify the presentation of the information, drug interaction information was categorized into several classes.

Drug Interactions:

Class-1A Interactions describe interactions that are based on the therapeutic activity of the herb, and an additive effect (e.g. stronger clinical activity) can occur when used in combination with certain pharmaceutical drugs.

Class-1B Interactions describe interactions that are based on the known active ingredients of the herb and that an additive effect (e.g. stronger clinical activity) can occur when used in combination with certain pharmaceutical drugs.

Class-2 Interactions describe effects that may occur when taking the herb and that are based on concerns arising from laboratory based experimental studies.

Class-3 Interactions describe interactions that are based on events that occurred in patients.

Class-4 Interactions describe the potential for the herb to induce or inhibit the cytochrome P450 metabolizing enzymes.

Note: **Class-1A** and **-1B interactions** are theoretical, in that an actual additive effect will occur only if the dosage of the active ingredients of the herb is at levels sufficient in your body. You should provide this information to your health-care practitioner, so that he is aware of this potential interaction.

Note: **Class-2 interactions** have not been observed in humans. Despite this, you should share this information with your health-care practitioner, as many side effects occur at very low incidents, and it may simply be a question of number of people having taken the herb before the incident is observed. It is better to be aware of these and to consult a health-care practitioner, if you believe that you are experiencing an effect that is possibly related to this activity.

Note: **Class-3 interactions** have been observed in people. You should ask your health-care practitioner about these if you have any concerns.

Note: **Class-4 interaction** information will be very important for your physician and/or pharmacist if you are taking any pharmaceutical medications. Cytochrome P450 enzymes are involved in the metabolism and are responsible for eliminating compounds from your body. If a product inhibits these enzymes, the result may be an increase in the level of a drug in your blood, and this could result in side effects. This is because there are fewer enzymes available in your body to remove the drug from the blood. As you continue to take the pill, the level of the drug continues to increase in your blood and, at one point, side effects will begin to appear. There are cases of serious side effects, including death, resulting from the increase in blood levels of a drug. The opposite is also possible, if the herb induces (e.g. activates the creation of more of these enzymes) these P450 enzymes. The result is that there are more enzymes available to remove the drug from the blood. The danger in this case is that less drug may be available to help cure your disease. A good example is with antibiotics. If the dose of the antibiotic in your blood is lower because of the P450 enzymes, then the infection can persist.

MONOGRAPH – BLACK COHOSH
(*Cimicifuga racemosa*)

Black cohosh (*Cimicifuga racemosa*), also known as **Black snakeroot**, has a long history of use with Native Indians in the treatment of pain and menstrual disorders. It was first used as a medicine in 1831 for the treatment of rheumatism, neuralgia, dysmenorrhea, as well as other non-pain conditions (Culbreth 1927). The medicinal drug Macrotys was prepared from the plant Black cohosh and was launched in Eclectic medicine in 1844 as a remedy for acute rheumatism and neuralgia (Felter 1922). It had many clinical indications for use including the treatment of rheumatoid and myalgic pain, as well as several conditions involving the reproductive organs of women (Felter 1922). Over time, it developed a reputation as an excellent remedy/anodyne (relieves pain) for rheumatoid pain (Felter 1922; Ellingwood & Lloyd 1919). This medicine was thought to possess sedative, cardiac, anodyne and antispasmodic properties. According to other authors, remedies have traditionally been used for the treatment of premenstrual and menopausal problems associated with neurovegetative complaints (van Wyk & Wink 2010), rheumatism, chorea, dizziness and tinnitus.

The active parts of the plant are the dried rhizome and roots. Doses range from 0.4 to 2.4 grams of the dried rhizome and/or root per day.

SAFETY: (van Wyk & Wink 2010; Natural Standard database; Health Canada)

According to a review study by Borrelli et al (2003) and studies by Lupu et al (2003), Black cohosh does not have estrogenic activity. The researchers suggested that this herb acts on the central nervous system instead of via a hormonal effect. A study by Seidlova-Wuttke et al (2003) supports the theory that Black cohosh does not have direct estrogenic activity and demonstrated that the herb acted on the hypothalamus/pituitary glands and on the bone but not directly on the uterus. The study by Reame et al (2008) examined changes in Luteinizing hormone pulsing and mu-opioid (mu or μ-opioid receptors refers to a type of receptor in our body) receptor binding activity in postmenopausal women. After 11 weeks of treatment with the herb, spontaneous pulsatile Luteinizing hormone secretion was unchanged compared to baseline. Their research demonstrated a lack of estrogenic action on the Hypothalamus-Pituitary-Ovarian axis. The results of their study demonstrated the neurobiological effects of the herb and that it acted on systems relevant to the pathophysiology of hot flashes. Since the herb does act on the hypothalamus/pituitary glands, caution should be taken with certain medical conditions, such as hormone-dependent cancer. In addition, based on our current knowledge of the herb, the use of this herb during pregnancy and breastfeeding should be avoided, due to potential effects of the active ingredients on the hypothalamus/pituitary glands of the fetus or babies.

According to Mahady et al (2008), regulatory agencies in Australia, Canada, and the European Union are concerned about a potential link between the use of this herb and liver toxicity. The expert committee of the US Pharmacopeia examined the reports (approximately thirty reports) regarding incidents of liver damage and, in all cases, the toxicities had been assigned a risk category of possible association. None of the thirty incidents were given a probable or certain risk category. According to these experts, the toxicological information did not reveal negative information about the herb. However, as a cautionary measure, these experts recommended that Black cohosh products should be labeled with a warning of a potential risk, if you have a liver disorder or develop symptoms of liver trouble (such as fatigue, weakness, loss of appetite, jaundice) during use.

Contraindications or Precautions:

Avoid this plant if you are allergic to salicylates (e.g. salicylic acid) or plants from the Ranunculaceae family (e.g. buttercup).

Do not use during pregnancy or while breast-feeding. According to Dugoua et al 2006, Black cohosh should be avoided during the first two trimesters of pregnancy because of its potential menstrual flow stimulating activity. In addition, based on its demonstrated effects on the hypothalamus-pituitary glands, you should avoid taking this herb during pregnancy.

Consult your physician prior to using if you:
- are suffering from hormone-dependent cancer or prior to using if you are taking tamoxifen (Nolvadex™, Istubal™, and Valodex™) or raloxifene (Evista™); or
- are taking hormone replacement therapy; or
- have a liver disorder or develop symptoms of liver trouble.

Bring a copy of the information contained in this herb monograph when you go see your physician or pharmacist. They may not be familiar with the recent scientific data concerning the safety of Black cohosh.

Drug Interactions:
Class-1A Interactions

The following potential interactions are based on the therapeutic activity of the herb, and an additive effect (e.g. stronger clinical activity) can occur when used in combination with certain pharmaceutical drugs. Additive effects can occur with the following classes of drugs:
- Analgesics
- Anti-inflammatory agents

Class-1B Interactions

The following potential interactions are based on the known active ingredients of the herb and an additive effect (e.g. stronger clinical activity) can occur when used in combination with certain pharmaceutical drugs. Additive effects can occur with the following classes of drugs:
- The herb contains salicylic acid/salicylates. Therefore, the herb may increase the anti-platelet effects or anti-coagulation effects of drugs.

Class-2 Interactions

The following potential interactions are based on concerns derived from effects observed in animals or in laboratory studies:
- There are reports of a hypotensive effect in animals. Consult a health-care practitioner if your blood pressure drops when taking Black cohosh along with your hypertension medication.
- A study demonstrated the effect of Black cohosh on human osteoblasts. This suggests that the herb can have a benefit on the skeletal system (e.g. bones) (Volker et al 2005).

Class-3 Interactions

The following potential interactions have been observed in patients:
- A clinical study demonstrated a better response in perimenopause mood symptoms when the herb was used with St. John's wort (Briese et al 2007).

Class-4 Interactions

According to experimental studies, Black cohosh does not appear to have a clinically relevant effect on the cytochrome P450 metabolizing enzymes 2D6 and 3A activity (Natural Standard database; Health Canada).

MONOGRAPH – BLACK CURRANT
(*Ribes nigrum*)

Black currant (*Ribes nigrum*) is commonly used in Europe as an anti-inflammatory remedy. This species is different from the **Northern Black currant** (*Ribes hudsonianum*) that is native to North America. Northern Black currant was used by Native Americans for treating colds and coughs, as well as other non-pain conditions (Marles et al 2000).

The active parts of the plants *Ribes nigrum* are the leaves, but the fruit and seeds have also been used for other applications. According to van Wyk & Wink (2010), remedies made from the leaves were used to treat arthritis, rheumatism, spasmodic cough and diarrhea. The seeds have mainly been used as an alternative to evening primrose oil, as it contains 15% gamma-linolenic acid. These remedies have a mild diuretic effect on patients. Doses range from 2 to 4 grams of dried leaves taken orally several times a day.

SAFETY: (van Wyk & Wink 2010; Natural Standard database)

Contraindications or Precautions:

Avoid products containing this herb if you are allergic to Black currant or other plants in the Saxifragaceae family.

Consult a health-care practitioner if you have a venous disorder. In a clinical trial in humans, this plant has been shown to increase peripheral blood flow and circulation in women with vein insufficiency (Allaert et al 1992).

Some people may experience diarrhoea and/or other symptoms related to the gastrointestinal tract. Therefore, use with caution if you have a gastrointestinal disorder.

Drug Interactions:
Class-1A Interactions

The following potential interactions are based on the therapeutic activity of the herb, and an additive effect (e.g. stronger clinical activity) can occur when used in combination with certain pharmaceutical drugs. Additive effects can occur with the following classes of drugs:
- Immune-modulators
- Anti-inflammatory agents
- Antithrombotic agents

Class-1B Interactions

The following potential interactions are based on the known active ingredients of the herb, and an additive effect (e.g. stronger clinical activity) can occur when used in combination with certain pharmaceutical drugs. Additive effects can occur with the following classes of drugs:
- This plant may have an additive effect with anticoagulants. Consult a health-care practitioner prior to use if you have haemophilia or if you are taking anticoagulants.
- According to the Natural Standard database, Black currant may have MAOI activity. Consult a health-care practitioner prior to use if you are taking monoamine oxidase inhibitors (MAOIs).

MONOGRAPH – BOSWELLIA
(*Boswellia sacra or serrata*)

Boswellia (*Boswellia sacra or serrata*), also known as Frankincense tree, is well known for its anti-inflammatory and analgesic properties. According to van Wyk & Wink (2010) "its resin has been used since ancient times for religious and medicinal purposes." It is also known for its expectorant properties and has been used externally to treat rheumatic conditions and internally to treat asthma. The active part of the plant is the resin.

The inhibition of 5-lipoxygenase has been proposed as a path for its beneficial effects in arthritis.

SAFETY: (van Wyk & Wink 2010; Natural Standard database; Health Canada)

Drug Interactions:
Class-1A Interactions

The following potential interactions are based on the therapeutic activity of the herb, and an additive effect (e.g. stronger clinical activity) can occur when used in combination with certain pharmaceutical drugs. Additive effects can occur with the following classes of drugs:
- Analgesics
- Anti-inflammatory agents

Class-2 Interactions

The following potential interactions are based on concerns derived from effects observed in animals or on laboratory studies.

- An experimental study suggested taking large amounts of Boswellia as it may induce liver toxicity (Kiela et al 2005).
- The resin of boswellia has been shown to lower cholesterol and triglyceride blood levels in rats (Natural Standard database).

Class-4 Interactions

According on experimental studies, the active ingredients (e.g. boswellic acids) of the herb are significant inhibitors of the Cytochrome P450 enzymes 1A2/2C8/2C9/ 2C19/2D6 and 3A4 (Frank and Unger 2006).

MONOGRAPH – BURDOCK
(*Arctium lappa*)

Burdock (*Arctium lappa*), also known as **Greater Burdock**, is an herb commonly used in North America, Europe and Asia. The active part of the plant is the dried root. The roots have traditionally been used to treat gastrointestinal disorders. The remedies have diuretic properties, and naturopathic medicine considers this as an emunctories draining herb. According to Culbreth (1927), it was used as a medicine for rheumatism and gout, as well as several other non-pain conditions.

SAFETY: (van Wyk & Wink 2010; Natural Standard database; Health Canada)

Contraindications or Precautions:

Avoid products containing this herb if you are allergic to burdock or members of the Asteraceae/Compositae family (e.g. ragweed, chrysanthemums, marigolds, and daisies). Parts of Burdock contain pectin so avoid using this plant if you have intolerance to pectin.

Drug Interactions:
Class-2 Interactions

The following potential interactions are based on concerns derived from effects observed in animals or on laboratory studies:
- Do not use during pregnancy, especially during the first trimester, due to the potential oxytocic and uterine stimulant activities of ingredients contained in Burdock (Natural Standard database).

- Consult a health-care practitioner prior to use if you are a diabetic, or are taking medication for diabetes. According to the Natural Standard database, Burdock may have hypoglycemic effects.

Class-3 Interactions

The following potential interactions have been observed in patients:
- Consult a health-care practitioner prior to use if you are taking diuretics. A diuretic effect was observed in patients (Natural Standard database).

MONOGRAPH – CALIFORNIA POPPY
(*Eschscholzia californica*)

California poppy (*Eschscholzia californica*) is an herb traditionally used in North America for its analgesic, hypnotic and sedative properties. The active part of the plant is the dried aerial parts. It has been traditionally used to treat sleeplessness (e.g. insomnia) in adults and children, anxiety, minor nervous disturbances, neuralgic pains, toothaches, and liver and gallbladder complaints (van Wyk & Wink 2010).

You may experience drowsiness when taking this herb. In the morning or during the day, if taking this herb, be very careful if you are using heavy machinery, driving a motor vehicle or involved in activities requiring mental alertness. You may also develop tolerance to the sensation of drowsiness after taking several doses of of this herb; however, in general you should continue to benefit from the hypnotic (e.g. sleep aid) effects of the herb. In general, people do not have a next-morning residual drowsiness when using this herb as a sleep aid. Also, there are no reports of reduced concentration or reduced motor coordination.

California poppy is known to contain the following alkaloids californidine; escholtzine; protopine; N-methyl-laurotetanine; caryachine; O-methylcaryachine; 6S,12S-neocaryachine-7-O-methyl ether N-metho salt , aporphine alkaloid.

Other experimental studies have confirmed the following pharmacological properties of California poppy (Gafner et al 2006; Rolland et al 2001): sedative, spasmolytic, anxiolytic and analgesic activities. According to other studies, the time it takes to fall asleep is reduced and the sleep quality is improved.

There is no known dependence or addiction to California poppy. This is why it is not classified as a narcotic or controlled drug.

Doses range from 0.5 to 3 grams per day of the dried herb.

SAFETY: (van Wyk & Wink 2010; Health Canada)

Contraindications or Precautions:

Avoid products containing this herb if you are allergic to California poppy (*Eschscholzia californica*) or related members of the Papaveraceae family. Also avoid these products if you are allergic to morphine, hydromorphone, codeine or derivatives of the same class.
The herb has anxiolytic therapeutic activity and may have a hypotensive effect when used in combination with other opioid analgesics and/or hypertensive medications.
There is no clinical data supporting the safe use in children and adolescents. Do not use during pregnancy.
There is a low incidence of people reporting insomnia subsequent to the use of California poppy extracts.

Drug Interactions:
Class-1A Interactions

The following potential interactions are based on the therapeutic activity of the herb, and an additive effect (e.g. stronger clinical activity) can occur when used in combination with certain pharmaceutical drugs. Additive effects can occur with the following classes of drugs:
- Analgesics
- Sedatives or tranquilizers

Class-1B Interactions

The following potential interactions are based on the known active ingredients of the herb, and an additive effect (e.g. stronger clinical activity) can occur when used in combination with certain pharmaceutical drugs. Additive effects can occur with the following classes of drugs:
- Antidepressants of the following classes: Mono-amine oxidase inhibitors (MAOIs), Selective Serotonin Reuptake Inhibitors (SSRIs) or Serotonin Norepinephrine Reuptake Inhibitors (SNRIs).

Class-3 Interactions

The following potential interactions have been observed in patients:
- Sedation
- Although the majority of people obtain a mild sedative effect, a small percentage of people that take California poppy experience insomnia.

Class-4 Interactions

According to experimental studies, California poppy should not cause a significant effect on the cytochrome P450 metabolizing enzyme 3A activity.

In vitro studies were performed using pure synthetic forms of the known ingredients of California poppy. These studies revealed that one of the alkaloids, Escholtzine, had strong inhibition of cytochrome P450 metabolizing enzyme 3A activity. The other alkaloids only had weak inhibition.

MONOGRAPH – CORYDALIS
(*Corydalis yanhusuo*)

Corydalis (*Corydalis yanhusuo*) is an herb used in Chinese medicine. In traditional Chinese medicine, it is used for its analgesic activity in treating "organ pain and pain of injury" (Bone 1996). The active part of the plant is the rhizome. Its analgesic and sedative properties have been demonstrated, and experimentally, it was shown that its active ingredients have potency equivalent to that of 40% of morphine (Bone 1996). One of its alkaloids, Tetrahydro-palmatine (THP), has a naloxone-resistant analgesic action and it had no affinity for opiate receptors. Its analgesic activity has been linked to other pain receptor systems such as dopamine, and its analgesic effects included treatment of neuralgia, dys-menorrhoea and headaches. Bone (1996) reported that tolerance develops but only at half the rate for morphine, that THP is non-addictive, and that the herb can be used to treat "any type of pain, in appropriate combinations, but especially visceral pain." It has also been used in the treatment of insomnia.

Doses range from 5 to 10 grams of the dried rhizome per day.

SAFETY: (WHO 1999)

Contraindications or Precautions:

Avoid products containing this herb if you are allergic to Corydalis or plants in the Fumariaceae or Papaveraceae family.

Because the herb has cytotoxic properties, it is contraindicated for use in during pregnancy and breast-feeding (WHO 1999).

It may cause drowsiness.

Drug Interactions:
Class-1A Interactions

The following potential interactions are based on the therapeutic activity of the herb, and an additive effect (e.g. stronger clinical activity) can occur when used in combination with certain pharmaceutical drugs. Additive effects can occur with the following classes of drugs:
- Analgesics
- Sedatives or tranquilizers

Class-1B Interactions

The following potential interactions are based on the known active ingredients of the herb, and an additive effect (e.g. stronger clinical activity) can occur when used in combination with certain pharmaceutical drugs. Additive effects can occur with the following classes of drugs:
- Antidepressants of the following classes: Monoamine oxidase inhibitors (MAOIs), Selective Serotonin Reuptake Inhibitors (SSRIs) or Serotonin Norepinephrine Reuptake Inhibitors (SNRIs).
- Sedatives / Hypnotics
- Antiarrhythmic
- Cytotoxic or antineoplastic

MONOGRAPH – DEVIL'S CLAW
(*Harpagophytum procumbens*)

Devil's claw (*Harpagophytum procumbens*) is a South African plant that is recognized for its anti-inflammatory properties. The active part of the plant is the dried secondary roots. It is considered a bitter tonic and an anti-inflammatory, antirheumatic and analgesic remedy. Today it is very popular for its use in the treatment of rheumatism and arthritis. According to van Wyk & Wink (2010), it has been traditionally used as a tonic, for digestive conditions and to treat pain, during and after labour.

Doses range from 0.6 to 9 grams of the dried root daily and can be taken as infusions (or the equivalent in the form of a dried extract) of 1 to 3 grams per dose.

There have been over 20 clinical trials with this herbal remedy showing benefits in low back pain, osteoarthritis and rheumatoid arthritis. The iridoid glycosides (e.g. harpagoside) have been linked to its anti-inflammatory and analgesic benefits.

SAFETY: (van Wyk & Wink 2010; Natural Standard database; Health Canada)

Contraindications or Precautions:

Avoid products containing this herb if you are allergic to Devil's claw (*Harpagophytum procumbens*). Common allergic side effects include diarrhea.

Based on traditional herbal practice, it is recommended to avoid taking if you have gastric or duodenal ulcers.

Drug Interactions:
Class-1A Drug Interactions

The following potential interactions are based on the therapeutic activity of the herb, and an additive effect (e.g. stronger clinical activity) can occur when used in combination with certain pharmaceutical drugs. Additive effects can occur with the following classes of drugs:
- Analgesics
- Non-Steroidal Anti-Inflammatory Drugs (NSAIDs)

Class-2 Interactions

The following concern is derived from effects observed in animals or in laboratory studies:
- You should consult your health practitioner prior to taking this herb, if you suffer from arrhythmias or are taking antiarrhythmic agents. This herb has been found to decrease myocardial contractility in animal studies.

MONOGRAPH – FEVERFEW
(*Chrysanthemum parthenium*)

Feverfew (*Chrysanthemum parthenium*) is a well-known herb for its benefits in the prevention of migraine headaches. The active parts of the plant are the aerial parts. It has been traditionally used to treat migraine, fever, rheumatic and skin conditions as well as gynaecological disorders (van Wyk & Wink 2010).

Doses range from 50 to 200 mg of dried leaves per day.

SAFETY: (van Wyk & Wink 2010; Natural Standard database; Health Canada)

Contraindications or Precautions:

Do not take if you are allergic to Feverfew (Chrysanthemum parthenium) or its constituent parthenolide or to members of the Asteraceae (Compositae) family. This herb may cause allergic reactions in people allergic to ragweed, chrysanthemums, daisies, and marigolds.

The oral consumption of the dried leaf of Feverfew (Chrysanthemum parthenium) has been shown to cause aphthous ulcers, lip and tongue irritation, mouth inflammation and ulceration. It is safer to use encapsulated products.

If you have been taking Feverfew (Chrysanthemum parthenium) for several weeks or more, do not suddenly stop taking this herb, as there is a risk of Feverfew withdrawal. The withdrawal symptoms include headache (rebound headache), anxiety, sleep disturbances, muscle stiffness, and muscle pain.

According to the historical use by herbalists, this herb may have abortifacient effects. Therefore, avoid taking this herb when pregnant or when trying to become pregnant.

Drug Interactions:
Class-1A Interactions

The following potential interactions are based on the therapeutic activity of the herb, and an additive effect (e.g. stronger clinical activity) can occur when used in combination with certain pharmaceutical drugs. Additive effects can occur with the following classes of drugs:
- Non-Steroidal Anti-Inflammatory Drugs (NSAIDs)
- Abortifacient drugs
- Aspirin

Class-2 Interactions

The following concern is derived from effects observed in animals or on laboratory studies:
- This is herb inhibits the serotonin 5-HT receptor that is involved in the treatment of migraine headaches. Based on theoretical concerns, this herb may affect the symptoms of depression or reduce the effectiveness of antidepressants. Therefore, talk to your health-care practitioner prior to using this herb, if you have depression or are taking antidepressant drugs.

MONOGRAPH – FIGWORT
(*Scrophularia nodosa*)

Figwort (*Scrophularia nodosa*), also known as **Common Figwort**, is a "forgotten" plant. Despite its long traditional history of use, this herb has been overlooked as a remedy for the treatment of pain and other conditions. The active plant parts are the dried aerial parts. It used to be well known for its anti-inflammatory and analgesic benefits, as well as its dermatological properties. It obtained its name from the traditional use of this plant against scrofula, which is a form of tuberculosis affecting the lymph nodes (van Wyk & Wink 2010). van Wyk & Wink (2010) stated "according to the *doctrine of signatures*, the nodular rhizomes resemble swollen lymph glands, thereby indicating that the plant may be effective in treating swellings and swollen glands."

There are about 200 species of Scrophularia including *Scrophularia nodosa* (Common Figwort) and *Scrophularia marilandica* (Late Figwort). Some refer to both of these plants as the same, and the name Carpenter's Square has been associated to both species of Scrophularia.

Doses range from 2 to 8 grams of the dried herb taken as an infusion or equivalent quantities in forms of extracts or tinctures taken daily.

Figwort is good for mild-to-moderate knee pain and is a very good herb for reducing swelling and inflammation of the joints, such as the knee.

This herb contains several iridoid glycosides including harpagoside, harpagide, aucubin, catapol and procumbide giving it a composition similar to that of Devil's claw. Some of these ingredients have well established anti-inflammatory properties.

SAFETY: (van Wyk & Wink 2010)

Contraindications or Precautions:

Do not use if you have heart conditions, diabetes, are pregnant or breastfeeding.

Avoid products containing Figwort if you are allergic to Devil's claw (*Harpagophytum procumbens*). The reason for this warning is that Figwort contains many ingredients that are similar to Devil's claw. Gastrointestinal side effects, such as diarrhea, are a common allergic side effect.

You should consult your health practitioner prior to taking this herb if you suffer from arrhythmias or are taking antiarrhythmic agents. This precaution is based on the fact that Devil's claw has been found to decrease myocardial contractility in animal studies.

Drug Interactions:
Class-1A Interactions

The following potential interactions are based on the therapeutic activity of the herb, and an additive effect (e.g. stronger clinical activity) can occur when used in combination with certain pharmaceutical drugs. Additive effects can occur with the following classes of drugs:
- Analgesics
- Non-Steroidal Anti-Inflammatory Drugs (NSAIDs)

MONOGRAPH – HORSETAIL
(*Equisetum arvense*)

Horsetail (*Equisetum arvense*), also known as **Field Horsetail**, is an herb commonly used in North America, Europe and Asia for its diuretic effects (van Wyk & Wink 2010). According to Marles et al (2000), Native Americans used to heat the root and placed it against the teeth to treat the pain. Its main use by Native Americans was a diuretic for kidney disorders. The active part of the plant is the dried stems and according to van Wyk & Wink (2010), it is used "as a diuretic to treat inflammation of the lower urinary tract, kidney gravel and post-traumatic and static oedema". This herb also has external uses for wound healing.

Doses range from 2 to 6 grams of the dried herb per day. This plant is well known as a source of silicon since it contains 5-8% silicic acid (van Wyk & Wink 2010).

SAFETY: (van Wyk & Wink 2010; Natural Standards database)

Contraindications or Precautions:

Avoid products containing Horsetail if you are allergic to *Equisetum arvense*, its constituents, or members of the Equisetaceae family.

When taking this herb, some people have had gastrointestinal symptoms, such as abdominal distension, increased frequency of bowel movements, and nausea.

There are safety concerns associated with the use of Horsetail in people that have cardiac arrhythmias or are taking antiarrhythmic agents (such as digoxin) or cardiac glycosides. Therefore, consult your health practitioner prior to use.

Use cautiously in patients with neurological disorders or in patients with thiamine deficiency, malnutrition or alcoholism. Depleting the body's thiamine could cause irreversible neurologic damage.

Drug Interactions:
Class-1A Interactions

The following potential interactions are based on the therapeutic activity of the herb, and an additive effect (e.g. stronger clinical activity) can occur when used in combination with certain pharmaceutical drugs. Additive effects can occur with the following classes of drugs:
- Diuretics
- Non-Steroidal Anti-Inflammatory Drugs (NSAIDs)

MONOGRAPH – LICORICE
(*Glycyrrhiza glabra*)

Licorice (liquorice) (Glycyrrhiza glabra) is not as well-known in western herbology for its antispasmodic effects in pain management. It is better known for its anti-inflammatory effects on the gastrointestinal tract and as an expectorant. According to van Wyk & Wink (2010), it has been used orally since ancient time to treat gastritis, epigastric bloating, flatulence, and coughs. It also has external uses for skin conditions. This plant is found in the *Eclectic Materia Medica*, but it had no recognized use in the treatment of pain conditions (Felter 1922). Ellingwood & Lloyd (1919) described that it was a useful demulcent for use in the treatment of inflammation of the lungs. The active plant part is the dried rhizome. The rhizome has been used externally for its anti-inflammatory properties.

An infusion made from 1 to 1.5 grams of the dried rhizome in 150 ml of boiling water is the common daily dose. According to WHO (1999), 5 to 15 grams of the dried plant material can be taken daily, and this corresponds to 200-800 mg of glycyrrhizin.

It has been used in Traditional Chinese medicine (TCM) for its antispasmodic activity. In fact it is commonly used in TCM in combination with White Peony for treating many types of muscle spasms, including those of the lower limbs. Its spasmolytic activity has been demonstrated in animals (WHO 1999).

Researchers have associated its anti-inflammatory properties to the corticosteroid-like activity of its ingredients glycyrrhizin and glycyrrhetic acid (WHO 1999).

SAFETY: (WHO 1999; van Wyk & Wink 2010; Natural Standard database; Health Canada)

Contraindications or Precautions:

Do not take if you are allergic to licorice, its constituents, or to members of the Fabaceae (Leguminaceae) family (pea family).

Many of the side effects of licorice are due to glycyrrhizic acid. These side effects are not expected to occur with *Deglycyrrhizinated licorice* (DGL). Taking excessive amounts of licorice may induce a type of mineralocorticoid excess syndrome. According to the Natural Standard database, this syndrome may cause hypokalemia, hypernatremia, metabolic alkalosis, fluid retention, and suppression of the renin-angiotensin-aldosterone system.

The most common side effects associated with Licorice are sodium retention and hypertension (Natural Standard database). When consumed in large amounts (e.g. over 50 grams per day), licorice has caused cardiac arrhythmias and ventricular tachycardia.

It is contraindicated for use in patients with hypertension, cholestatic disorders or cirrhosis of the liver, hypokalemia, or chronic renal insufficiency, and during pregnancy (WHO 1999).

Drug Interactions:
Class-1A Interactions

The following potential interactions are based on the therapeutic activity of the herb, and an additive effect (e.g. stronger clinical activity) can occur when used in combination with certain pharmaceutical drugs. Additive effects can occur with the following classes of drugs:

- Based on its corticosteroid-like activity, do not use when taking corticosteroids.
- Licorice causes an increased elimination of potassium. Therefore, consult your health-care practitioner prior to use when taking thiazide, loop diuretics or cardiac glycosides.

Class-3 Interactions

The following potential interactions have been observed in patients:
- There are several cases of acute myopathy (e.g. muscle injury) following the long term use of licorice (Natural Standard database).

Class-4 Interactions

According on experimental studies, constituents of licorice have been shown to inhibit the cytochrome P450 enzyme.

MONOGRAPH – MEADOWSWEET
(*Filipendula ulmaria*)

Meadowsweet (*Filipendula ulmaria*), also known as **queen-of-the-meadow**, is an herb commonly used in Europe and Asia for treating pain. The pharmaceutical drug Aspirin™ was named after *Spiraea ulmaria* which is the old name for Meadowsweet (van Wyk & Wink 2010). The active part of the plant that is traditionally used is the dried flower or dried aerial part of the plant. Remedies made from this plant are considered both anti-inflammatory and analgesic.

This plant should not be mistaken for **Queen of the Meadow,** which is also known as **Gravel root,** (*Eupatorium purpureum*).

Meadowsweet remedies are used in the treatment of arthritis and rheumatism as well as colds for its antipyretic (e.g. reduce fever) properties (van Wyk & Wink 2010).

Doses range from 2.5 to 3.5 grams of the dried flower or 4 to 5 grams of the dried herb per day.

SAFETY: (van Wyk & Wink 2010; Natural Standard database)

Contraindications or Precautions:

Do not take if you are allergic to salicylates or aspirin or if you are allergic to Meadowsweet, *Filipendula* spp. and other members of the Roseaceae family.

This herb may worsen asthma. If this occurs, it may be due to the presence of the aspirin triad, a common co-occurrence of asthma, rhinitis, and aspirin allergy (Natural Standard database).

Avoid use in infants with fever due to the risk of Reye's syndrome (e.g. Reye's syndrome is associated with the consumption of salicylates).

When taken in large amounts, gastric and renal irritation, hypersensitivity, nausea and vomiting, and tinnitus can occur due to the salicylate content of the herb.

Avoid taking Meadowsweet during pregnancy:
- Meadowsweet may increase uterine tone and might stimulate uterine activity.
- Avoid taking during the third trimester since salicylates can lead to premature closure of the ductus arteriosus and induce cardiac and pulmonary abnormalities in the fetus (Natural Standard database).

Class-1A Interactions

The following potential interactions are based on the therapeutic activity of the herb, and an additive effect (e.g. stronger clinical activity) can occur when used in combination with certain pharmaceutical drugs. Additive effects can occur with the following classes of drugs:
- Analgesic
- Anti-inflammatory
- Anticoagulant: can increase the risk of bleeding
- Antiplatelet: can increase the risk of bleeding
- Antipyretic
- Muscle relaxants: Meadowsweet has muscle relaxant activity

MONOGRAPH – SKULLCAP
(*Scutellaria lateriflora*)

Skullcap (*Scutellaria lateriflora*) (sometimes spelled Scullcap), also known as Virginia Skullcap and Helmet flower, is a well know anxiolytic and sedative herb. The active plant part is the dried aerial parts. It is known for its anticonvulsant, sedative, and antispasmodic properties. It should not be mistaken for its Asian sister (a well known Chinese herb) (Baical Skullcap / *Scutellaria baicalensis*) which are known for their anti-inflammatory, anti-allergic and circulatory properties.

Native Americans used Marsh Skullcap (*Scutellaria galericulata*) as a remedy for ulcers and fever (Marles et al 2000). According to these authors, an extract of Marsh Skullcap showed no sedative or antispasmodic effects. According to the *Eclectic Materia Medica* (Felter 1922), Skullcap is calmative to the nervous and muscular systems. Felter (1922) described it as able to control nervous irritability and muscular incoordination, thereby providing rest and allowing sleep, and it was described as a remedy for insomnia due to worry, nervous irritability or nervous excitability. It was used to control muscular twitching and tremors. Similar properties were described in the *American Materia Medica*, including the ability of the herb to induce a quiet and restful sleep via its action on the nervous system (Ellingwood & Lloyd 1919).

Virginia Skullcap was traditionally used as a nerve tonic and sedative including for its use in the treatment of epilepsy, grand mal, hysteria and nervous conditions (van Wyk & Wink 2010). According to Culbreth (1927), it was used as a nervine and antispasmodic medicine in the early 1900's and the *Manual of Materia Medica* lists the following pain associated conditions where it was used: spasms, muscular twitching, and neuralgia. Today it is widely used for treating tension, anxiety and insomnia as well as a visceral relaxant / antispasmodic for muscular cramps.

79

Typical doses range from infusion of 1 to 2 grams of the dried herb taken 3 times a day to equivalent amounts in the form of extracts or tinctures. You can take 0.25 to 12 grams of the dried herb top per day.

SAFETY: (van Wyk & Wink 2010; Natural Standard database; Health Canada)

Contraindications or Precautions:

Do not take if you are allergic to Scullcap (*Scutellaria lateriflora*), its constituents, or members of the Lamiaceae family.

Some people may experience drowsiness. Therefore, use caution if operating heavy machinery, driving a motor vehicle or involved in activities requiring mental alertness.

Consumption with alcohol, other drugs and/or natural health products with sedative properties is not recommended as an additive effect may occur.

Drug Interactions:
Class-1A Interactions

The following potential interactions are based on the therapeutic activity of the herb, and an additive effect (e.g. stronger clinical activity) can occur when used in combination with certain pharmaceutical drugs. Additive effects can occur with the following classes of drugs:
- Sedatives
- Tranquilizers
- Antidepressant agents
- Hypnotic drugs
- Anxiolytic agents

Class-2 Interactions

The following potential interactions are based on concerns derived from effects observed in animals or on laboratory studies.
- Based on an *in vitro* study, *Scutellaria lateriflora* may inhibit the 5-HT(7) serotonin receptor. The inhibition of this receptor is involved with anti-anxiety and antidepressant effects.

Class-3 Interactions

The following potential interactions have been observed in patients:
- Based on a double-blind, placebo controlled study, *Scutellaria lateriflora* was found to have an anti-anxiety effect in healthy people (Natural Standard database).

MONOGRAPH – STINGING NETTLE
(*Urtica dioica*)

Stinging nettle (*Urtica dioica*) is considered a weed by many, despite its established medicinal benefits. The active parts of the plant are both the aerial parts and the roots; however, each of these has different clinical benefits. For pain management, we use the aerial parts and for urological conditions the roots are used. The aerial parts of the plant have an established use in the treatment of rheumatic conditions.

Doses range from 8 to 12 grams daily of the dried leaves. According to van Wyk & Wink (2010), remedies made from the aerial part are anti-inflammatory and lower doses of pharmaceutical non-steroidal anti-inflammatory drugs are taken when these remedies are used concomitantly in the treatment of arthritis.

Native Americans used Stinging nettle as a remedy for diarrhea, intestinal worms, male urinary problems, asthma and as a blood purifier (Marles et al 2000). The *Eclectic Materia Medica* and *American Materia Medica* did not recognize its use for treating pain (Felter 1922; Ellingwood & Lloyd 1919).

SAFETY: (van Wyk & Wink 2010; Natural Standard database; Health Canada)

Contraindications or Precautions:

Do not take if you are allergic to Stinging Nettle, the Urticaceae family or any constituent of nettle products.

Mild gastric discomfort may occur when the herb is taken on an empty stomach. Other gastrointestinal side effects include constipation, diarrhea and gastric disorder.

Drug Interactions:
Class-1A Interactions

The following potential interactions are based on the therapeutic activity of the herb, and an additive effect (e.g. stronger clinical activity) can occur when used in combination with certain pharmaceutical drugs. Additive effects can occur with the following classes of drugs:
- Anti-inflammatory agents
- Analgesics

Class-3 Interactions

The following potential interactions have been observed in patients:
- In a clinical trial, Stinging nettle leaves plus diclofenac (50 mg) was as just effective in the treatment of acute arthritis as diclofenac 200 mg (Natural Standard database).

MONOGRAPH – TURMERIC
(*Curcuma longa*)

Turmeric (*Curcuma longa*) is a well-known herb in India where it is believed to have originated. Today this herb is well known in western herbology. The active part of the plant is the rhizomes and it is used for its choleretic and anti-inflammatory properties. According to van Wyk & Wink (2010), the rhizomes are used in treating peptic conditions including the stimulation of bile secretion and peptic ulcers. Although Turmeric appears in earlier material medica textbooks (Culbreth 1927), the pain management benefits of this herb were not recognized during this period.

Doses range from 2 to 9 grams of the dried rhizome daily.

Curcuminoids are recognized for their anti-inflammatory properties.

SAFETY: (van Wyk & Wink 2010; Natural Standard database; Health Canada)

Contraindications or Precautions:

Avoid products containing this herb if you are allergic to Turmeric ' (*Curcuma longa*), its ingredient curcumin or yellow food colorings, or other members of the Zingiberaceae (ginger) family.

Do not use in patients with obstruction of the bile duct or with gallstones.

Turmeric and curcumin are both considered safe even at relatively high dose levels (for example 6 grams). Despite its traditional reputation as a remedy for gastrointestinal disorders, its common side effects are gastrointestinal. Consult your health-care practitioner prior to use if you have stomach ulcers or disorder of the gastrointestinal tract.

Although clinical data has not shown an effect of turmeric on the absorption of iron, it is recommended that you do not take iron supplements at the same time. It is better to wait 2 hours between the turmeric and iron supplement. This concern is based on animal studies that demonstrated that turmeric may reduce the absorption of iron.

This herb has high oxalate content. Therefore, talk to your health-care practitioner prior to use, if you have, or if you are at risk for developing kidney stones.

Drug Interactions:
Class-1A Interactions

The following potential interactions are based on the therapeutic activity of the herb, and an additive effect (e.g. stronger clinical activity) can occur when used in combination with certain pharmaceutical drugs. Additive effects can occur with the following classes of drugs:
- Non-Steroidal Anti-Inflammatory Drugs (NSAIDs)

Class-1B Interactions

The following potential interactions are based on the known active ingredients (e.g. curcuminoids) of the herb and that an additive effect (e.g. stronger clinical activity) can occur when used in combination with certain pharmaceutical drugs. Additive effects can occur with the following classes of drugs:
- Non-Steroidal Anti-Inflammatory Drugs (NSAIDs).

Class-4 Interactions

According on experimental studies, Turmeric (curcumin) is a potent inhibitor of cytochrome P450 (CYP) 1A1/1A2, a less potent inhibitor of CYP 2B1/2B2, and a weak inhibitor of CYP 2E1.

MONOGRAPH – VALERIAN
(*Valeriana officinalis*)

Valerian (*Valeriana officinalis*), also known as **Common Valerian**, is a popular sleep remedy. The active parts of the plant are the rhizomes and roots, and remedies made from these are considered sedatives (tranquilizers). It is a mild sedative and sleep-promoting agent and has been used as an alternative to pharmaceutical sedatives, such as benzo-diazepines in the treatment of nervous excitation and anxiety-induced sleep disturbances (WHO 1999). Its use as a sleep aid has been demonstrated in clinical trials. According to van Wyk & Wink (2010), it is recognized as a non-addictive tranquilizer for the treatment of restlessness, sleeplessness, minor nervous conditions, symptoms of menopause, and anxiety associated with premenstrual syndrome, and it has been traditionally used as supportive treatment for gastrointestinal pain and spastic colitis. Based on its antispasmodic properties, it has been used as an adjuvant in spasmolytic states of smooth muscle and gastrointestinal pains of nervous origin (WHO 1999).

In the early 1900's, it was listed as a medicine in the *American* and *Eclectic Materia Medica* and used for the following pain associated conditions: as an anodyne, nervine, antispasmodic (Culbreth 1927). Culbreth (1927) stated that when used continuously it could produce "melancholia". According to Marles et al (2000), this plant was used for multiple medical purposes by the Native Americans but none were for treating pain. The *Eclectic Materia Medica* described this plant as cerebral and spinal stimulant and a good calmative for nervousness (Felter 1922). The *American Materia Medica* (Ellingwood & Lloyd 1919) viewed the plant as a non-narcotic, recognized it as a nervine, and listed the following indications: hysterical conditions, nervous excitement, etc.

Doses range from 2 to 10 grams of the dried root daily taken in doses of 2 to 3 grams 1 to 5 times a day.

SAFETY: (WHO 1999; van Wyk & Wink 2010; Natural Standard database; Health Canada)

Contraindications or Precautions:

Do not take if you are allergic to Valerian or members of the Valerianaceae family.

The following side effects may occur: headache, excitability, insomnia, uneasiness, ataxia, and hypothermia.

According to Natural Standard database, short-term mild impairments in vigilance, concentration, and processing time for complex thoughts, as well as mild fatigue is possible when taking Valerian. However, the residual sedative effects appear to be less pronounced than those associated with benzo-diazepines.

It is contraindicated for use in during pregnancy and breastfeeding (WHO 1999). There is a potential teratogenic effect from the valepotriates content of the herb.

It may cause drowsiness.

One of its classes of ingredients, valepotriates, is considered a potential mutagen. According to van Wyk & Wink (2010), aqueous preparations are safer than alcoholic extracts.

Drug Interactions:
Class-1A Interactions

The following potential interactions are based on the therapeutic activity of the herb, and an additive effect (e.g. stronger clinical activity) can occur when used in combination with certain pharmaceutical drugs. Additive effects can occur with the following classes of drugs:

- Alcohol
- Analgesics including codeine
- Antidepressant drugs including monoamine oxidase inhibitors (MAOIs)
- Antihistamines such as diphenhydramine (Benadryl®)
- Antianxiety and antipsychotic drugs including Selective serotonin reuptake inhibitors (SSRI)
- Barbiturates and benzodiazepines
- Sedatives
- Tranquilizers
- Antispasmodics

Class-4 Interactions

Based on a clinical study (Natural Standard database), multiple night-time doses of valerian (*Valeriana officinalis*) had minimal effects on CYP3A4 activity and no effect on CYP2D6 activity in healthy volunteers.

MONOGRAPH – WHITE PEONY
(*Paeonia lactiflora*)

White Peony (*Paeonia lactiflora*) is an herb commonly used in India and Asia for its analgesic, anti-inflammatory and antispasmodic properties (van Wyk & Wink 2010; WHO 1999; Bone 1996). According to Bone 1996, it relieves spasms and is used in the treatment of muscle cramping and dysmenorrhoea. Experimental studies demonstrated these pharmacological properties.

It has been traditionally used in the treatment of headache, amenorrhea, dysmenorrhoea, and pain in the chest and abdomen, as well as lower limbs (e.g. spasms of the calf muscles) (WHO 1999). The active part of the plant that is traditionally used is the dried root.

The doses range from 6 to 15 grams of the dried root per day.

SAFETY: (WHO 1999; Natural Standard database)

Contraindications or Precautions:

Do not take if you are allergic to White Peony, its constituents, or members of the Paeoniaceae family.

Side effects may include nausea and vomiting.

White Peony should not be used during the first trimester of pregnancy and tree peony bark should not be used at all during pregnancy. Traditionally, White peony has been used as an abortifacient and emmenagogue (WHO 1999).

Drug Interactions:
Class-1A Drug Interactions

The following potential interactions are based on the therapeutic activity of the herb, and an additive effect (e.g. stronger clinical activity) can occur when used in combination with certain pharmaceutical drugs. Additive effects can occur with the following classes of drugs:
- Analgesic
- Anti-inflammatory
- Antispasmodics
- Muscle relaxants

Class-2 Interactions

The following potential interactions are based on concerns derived from effects observed in animals or on laboratory studies:
- An ingredient of the root of Peony was shown to dilate vascular smooth muscle and suppress the vascular inflammatory process.

MONOGRAPH – WHITE WILLOW
(*Salix alba*)

White Willow (*Salix alba*) is a species of willow native to Europe and Asia and is well known for its content of the active ingredient salicin. The active plant part is the dried willow bark from 2 to 3 year old branches (van Wyk & Wink 2010). This plant is well known for its anti-inflammatory, analgesic and antipyretic effects. Remedies have traditionally been used for the treatment of fever/flu, rheumatism, headaches and other minor pain. In the early 1900's, its use in treating acute rheumatism, fever, relieving pain, and neuralgia was recognized in the *Manual of Materia Medica* (Culbreth 1927).

Doses range from 2 to 3 grams of powdered bark in one cup of cold water and then heating to boiling. A cupful is taken 3 to 4 times per day.

The Native Americans used several species of willow for medicinal purposes: Bebb's willow (*Salix bebiana*), Blueberry willow (*Salix myrtillifolia*), Diamondleaf willow (*S. Planifolia*), Balsam willow (*S. Pyrifolia*), etc (Marles et al 2000). The bark of these species also contains different salicylates including salicin. The inner bark was used to treat toothaches, as well as various non-pain conditions.

The *American Materia Medica* (Ellingwood & Lloyd 1919) described its use in many non-pain conditions.

SAFETY: (WHO 1999; Natural Standard database)

Contraindications or Precautions:

Do not take if you are allergic to aspirin, willow bark (*Salix* spp.), salicylates or Meadowsweet.

Side effects may include gastrointestinal problems (diarrhea, heartburn, vomiting and dyspepsia) and headaches.

Salicylates are known to impair platelet function, resulting in an increased bleeding time. The combined use of aspirin and willow bark may increase the risk of bleeding due to an additive effect.

The concomitant use of NSAIDS with willow bark may increase the risk of stomach ulceration and bleeding due to the salicylate content of willow bark.

Drug Interactions:
Class-1A Interactions

The following potential interactions are based on the therapeutic activity of the herb, and an additive effect (e.g. stronger clinical activity) can occur when used in combination with certain pharmaceutical drugs. Additive effects can occur with the following classes of drugs:
- Anti-inflammatory agents
- Analgesics
- Anticoagulants
- Antiplatelet

Class-3 Interactions

The following potential interactions have been observed in patients in a clinical trial:
- Some patients had blood pressure instability and edema.

WORKS CITED

Allaert et al 1992. Allaert, F. A., Vin, F., and Levardon, M. *Comparative study of the effectiveness of continuous or intermittent courses of a phlebotonic drug on venous disorders disclosed or aggravated by oral, estrogen-progesterone contraceptives.* Phlebologie. 1992; 45(2):167-173.

Bone 1996. K Bone, *Clinical applications of Ayurvedic and Chinese herbs.* Phytotherapy Press, Australia, 1996.

Borrelli, F., Izzo, A. A., and Ernst, E. *Pharmacological effects of Cimicifuga racemosa.* Life Sci. 7-25-2003;73(10):1215-1229.

Briese et al 2007. Briese, V., Stammwitz, U., Friede, M., and Henneicke-von Zepelin, H. H. *Black cohosh with or without St. John's wort for symptom-specific climacteric treatment-results of a large-scale, controlled, observational study.* Maturitas 8-20-2007;57(4):405-414.

Culbreth 1927. D M R Culbreth, *A Manual of Materia Medica and Pharmacology.* Lea & Febiger, Philadelphia, 1927.

Dugoua et al 2006. Dugoua, J. J., Seely, D., Perri, D., Koren, G., and Mills, E. *Safety and efficacy of black cohosh (Cimicifuga racemosa) during pregnancy and lactation.* Can J Clin Pharmacol 2006;13(3):e257-e261.

Ellingwood & Lloyd 1919. Ellingwood F and Lloyd J U, *American Materia Medica, Therapeutics and Pharmacognosy.* Eclectic Medical Publications, Cincinnati, Ohio 1919.

Felter 1922. *The Eclectic Materia Medica, Pharmacology and Therapeutics.* Eclectic Medical Publications, Cincinnati, Ohio 1922.

Frank and Unger 2006. Frank, A. and Unger, M. *Analysis of frankincense from various Boswellia species with inhibitory activity on human drug metabolising cytochrome P450 enzymes using liquid chromatography mass spectrometry after automated on-line extraction.* J Chromatogr A 4-21-2006; 1112(1-2):255-262.

Gafner S et al 2006. Gafner S, Dietz BM, McPhail KL, Scott IM et al. *Alkaloids from Eschscholzia californica and their capacity to inhibit binding of [³H]8-hydroxy-2-(di-N-propylamino)tetralin to 5-HT₁ₐ receptors in vitro.* J Nat Prod 2006, 69, 432-435.

Grieve M 1971. Mrs. M Grieve. *A modern herbal: The medicinal, culinary, cosmetic and economic properties, cultivation and folk-lore of herbs, grasses, fungi, shrubs and trees with all their modern scientific uses.* Volumes I and II. Dover Publication, Inc, New York. 1971.

Health Canada. Monographs prepared by the Natural Health Products Directorate, Health Canada. http://webprod.hc-sc.gc.ca/nhpid-bdipsn/monosReq.do?lang=eng ; Accessed 2011.

Kiela et al 2005. Kiela, P. R., Midura, A. J., Kuscuoglu, N., Jolad, S. D., Solyom, A. M., Besselsen, D. G., Timmermann, B. N., and Ghishan, F. K. *Effects of Boswellia serrata in mouse models of chemically induced colitis.* Am J Physiol Gastrointest.Liver Physiol 2005;288(4):G798-G808.

Lupu et al 2003. Lupu, R., Mehmi, I., Atlas, E., Tsai, M. S., Pisha, E., Oketch-Rabah, H. A., Nuntanakorn, P., Kennelly, E. J., and Kronenberg, F. *Black cohosh, a menopausal remedy, does not have estrogenic activity and does not promote breast cancer cell growth.* Int J Oncol. 2003;23(5):1407-1412.

95

Mahady et al 2008. Mahady, G. B., Low, Dog T., Barrett, M. L., Chavez, M. L., Gardiner, P., Ko, R., Marles, R. J., Pellicore, L. S., Giancaspro, G. I., and Sarma, D. N. *United States Pharmacopeia review of the black cohosh' case reports of hepatotoxicity.* Menopause. 2008;15(4 Pt 1):628-638.

Marles et al 2000. Marles RJ, Clavelle C, Monteleone L, Tays N and Burns D, *Aboriginal plant use in Canada's Northwest Boreal Forest,* Natural Resources Canada, UBC Press, Vancouver 2000.

Moore et al 2003. Moore A, Edwards J, Barden J et McQuay H. *Bandolier's Little Book of Pain.* Oxford University Press, 2003.

Natural Standard database. *Evidence-based Systematic Reviews of herbs* by the Natural Standard Research Collaboration. Copyright ® 2011. www.natural standard.com. Accessed 2011.

Reame et al 2008. Reame, N. E., Lukacs, J. L., Padmanabhan, V., Eyvazzadeh, A. D., Smith, Y. R., and Zubieta, J. K. *Black cohosh has central opioid activity in postmenopausal women: evidence from naloxone blockade and positron emission tomography neuroimaging.* Menopause. 2008; 15(5):832-840.

Rolland A et al 2001. Rolland A, Fleurentin J, Lanhers MC et al. *Neurophysiological effects of an extract of Escholzia californica Cham (Papaveraceae).* Phytother. Res. 2001; 15:377-381.

Sarris J et Wardle J 2010. Sarris J et Wardle J. *Clinical naturopathy: an evidence-based guide to practice.* Churchill Livingstone, Elsevier. 2010.

Seidlova-Wuttke et al 2003. Seidlova-Wuttke, D., Hesse, O., Jarry, H., Christoffel, V., Spengler, B., Becker, T., and Wuttke, W. *Evidence for selective estrogen receptor modulator activity in a black cohosh (Cimicifuga racemosa) extract: comparison with estradiol-17beta.* Eur.J Endocrinol. 2003;149(4): 351-362.

van Wyk & Wink 2010. BE van Wyk and M Wink, *Medicinal Plants of the World*, Timber Press, 2010.

Viereck et al 2005. Viereck, V., Grundker, C., Friess, S. C., Frosch, K. H., Raddatz, D., Schoppet, M., Nisslein, T., Emons, G., and Hofbauer, L. C. *Isopropanolic extract of black cohosh stimulates osteoprotegerin production by human osteoblasts.* J Bone Miner. Res 2005;20(11):2036-2043.

WHO (1999). World Health Organization, Geneva. *WHO monographs on selected medicinal plants.* Volume 1, 1999.

ABOUT THE AUTHOR

GUY CHAMBERLAND, *M.Sc., Ph.D., Herbalist*, is a retired drug development specialist that spent over 15 years in the pharmaceutical industry bringing new products from discovery to *first in human* clinical trials and then to the market. He obtained a Master's of Science and Doctorate (PhD) degree in the biomedical sciences (field of toxicology). Chamberland developed an expertise in drug safety and regulatory affairs while working in the pharmaceutical and biotechnology industries.

Chamberland has completed training as a natural health practitioner, bioenergetics practitioner, chartered herbalist, in herbal prescriptions, and wrote a Master Herbalist thesis. Through his continued research in herbal science, he has become an expert in herbal pain management.

He founded the company called CuraPhyte Technologies. www.curaphyte.com and www.enteriphyte. com. You can reach Chamberland at gchamberland@ curaphyte.ca.

This book is available in e-book version. He is currently working on his next book entitled *Scientific Look at Herbal Remedies: Is there more than Traditional Evidence?*